Positive Pregnancy

What you CAN do to Support Your Pregnancy

Bernadette Connolly

BSc (Hons) Osteopathic Medicine

To my son:

Thank you for showing me what true love is and what it is to be a mother.

To my family & friends:

*Thank you for the support you have given me in my journey to help others
with my experiences.*

To the hedgefunder's wife:

*Thank you for giving me the inspiration to help women. I hope
you have found the peace you need to heal as a mother.*

Contents

Preface

In 2005, I found out I was having my first child and got to experience the UK's maternity services for myself. Being headstrong allowed me to ignore any fear mongering, but made me realise how terrifying pregnancy could be for other mums. The NCT classes seeming more like a analgesic sales pitch for pharmaceuticals than a pregnancy support group, based on our fear of the pain in labour. I stopped paying attention to the negativity and began to listen to myself, my body and my baby instead. I became aware of what my body was telling me. For example: my first craving was a vegetable with a very high amount of folate – sprouts! My body knew and once I began to listen, my pregnancy became a positive experience, regardless of personal issues I had at the time. This mindset was empowering and somewhat magical. Even after labour, I was in awe of my body respond to things before I was consciously aware of them. I honestly wish I could have bottled that feeling!

If you have read the ebook series you will know a little more about my personal experiences with NHS maternity servies, I feel it isnt worth wiriting here again but know that my experience opened my eyes to how flawed our maternity services are. These flaws are what motivated me to help women, and why I chose to specialise in pregnancy and post natal therapy during my time as an osteopath.

Nine months is a long time when growing and carrying new life, the last month by far the longest.

During the pandemic I treated the wife of a prestigous

hedgefunder in Surrey. They had left the hustle and bustle of London and moved to more a more peacful place. Sadly this lady was suffering with post partum depression and I was caught in the cross fire. However, this made me realise that even with stacks of money women need more support in pregenancy and postnatal care, and this inspired me to start my ebook series and now this book.

Introduction

L ife is full of surprises, some hoped for and others unplanned. Whether you had anticipated pregnancy or not, it can still be daunting not knowing what to expect in the next 9 months. Every pregnancy is different, some easier than others. If we ask friends and family about their experiences we are often given negative stories which can end up creating unnecessary fears in ourselves. Looking for information online will provide you with weekly updates about the baby's development, however, there isn't much written about the magnificent changes that your body is going through. Certain symptoms of pregnancy can also be looked up, but *Doctor Google* related stress isn't what you need right now.

The past few years have reduced public's confidence in the medical industry globally. The impact of the pandemic on health services has resulted in many seeking alternative therapies and self care techniques to avoid the lengthy waiting times. The UK's maternity services were forced to make thousands of women to give birth alone with minimal support, both during and after pregnancy. This has resulted in an increase in postnatal depression and a decrease in allocated support.

Having been a pregnancy and post natal osteopath for over 7 years, I worked with a number of expecting mothers and learned that not much has changed. The UK's maternity services seem to be stuck in an outdated approach towards pregnancy and child birth. Thankfully people are becoming more aware of the alternative antenatal choices, giving them more options and a sense of independence throughout their pregnancy.

It is normal to feel overwhelmed, even if this isn't your first pregnancy. Maternity advice has changed drastically over the past 20 years and what may have been considered helpful might now be considered unsafe.

Many women express concerns about advised limitations to both activities and foods, especially in the first trimester. These lifestyle changes can seem unfair, but healthcare professionals have a duty to outline potential risks in order to prevent avoidable complications. Feeling restricted as a result of advice from healthcare professionals is in fact a common cause for antenatal anxiety!

Antenatal anxiety is more common than we are told; especially for new mothers, those who have experienced a traumatic labour, or a loss. In a 2017 review of 102 studies involving over 220,000 women (Dennis et al, 2017), self-reported anxiety symptoms averaged at 18.2% in the first trimester, 19.1% in the second trimester and 24.6% in the third trimester. While these percentages may seem small, it's worth noting they are based on self-reported numbers and in reality many struggle without telling anyone. A large number of studies on antenatal mental health share the same conclusion that more research is needed to develop effective evidence-based interventions. While this is still being explored, alternative antenatal practices are leading the way by improving individual experiences and encouraging existing services to evolve.

From both personal and professional experience, I agree that there needs to be a positive change towards both pregnancy and parenthood. My awareness of this need is a large reason for this book and all others in the positive pregnancy series. My aim is to normalise treating pregnancy with the respect it deserves, supporting independent pregnancies, encouraging informed choices and making pregnancy a positively enjoyable experience. Providing details on activities, nutrition, exercises and support through each trimester allows you to choose what you want for your pregnancy instead of worrying about what you can't have.

While this is a pregnancy book in itself, unlike most it is focused on the mother's body instead of developmental stages of the baby and risk based restrictions. There are a plethora of pregnancy books out now which is wonderful, however, some books cause mothers to place unnecessary pressure on themselves which can lead to further issues in the long term.

NB: There is no perfect way to parent, its is a learning curve with each pregnancy (and baby) as no two are the same, not even twins! Your journey is yours alone so my strongest advice is to take what works for you and leave what does not.

How to use this book.

This book is organised it into four parts; one for each trimester of pregnancy and a final section discussing post natal recovery - also known as the fourth trimester. Each part has chapters about changes to your body during that time. Additionally there is information on exercises for each trimester, aimed at helping prevent commonly experienced symptoms. Each trimester also has nutritional advice as well as activities aimed at supporting your journey.

Reading each part separately breaks the book down in to manageable chunks and allows you to consider your options for each individual trimester. As you approach the last month of each trimester it is recommended to begin reading the next part. This helps you to plan ahead for any additional options you may (or may not) wish to add.

All of the suggestions given in this book are recommendations - not directions, each having an explanation for their inclusion. Your health advisor or midwife will advise you of things you should avoid so I have kept that to a minimum so you can concentrate on the things that you would like to include instead.

Please note:

If you are under observation for any reason, please consult your health professional before implementing any changes.

Part One

The First Trimester

The First Trimester

"You are the closest I will

ever come to magic."

- Suzanne Dunnamore

How you react to finding out you are pregnant varies for everyone - some mothers become excited, some apprehensive. Interestingly, both of these reactions come from the sympathetic nervous system which is known for your fight or flight response.

How you feel about your journey is another variable, however, being aware of what to expect and armed with informed choices will help make the journey easier.

For many women, the first trimester is accompanied by a range of symptoms such as morning sickness, fatigue, breast tenderness, and mood swings, as hormonal fluctuations take hold. These symptoms, while challenging, are often a reassuring sign of the pregnancy progressing as expected. Moreover, during the first trimester, prenatal care becomes paramount, with regular visits to healthcare providers for check-ups, screenings, and guidance on nutrition and lifestyle adjustments. Emotionally, the first trimester can be a time of excitement, anticipation, and perhaps some anxiety as the reality of impending parenthood sets in. Expectant parents may begin to share the news with family and friends, further cementing the bond with their growing baby. Overall, the first trimester is a period of significant change and adjustment, laying the foundation for the remarkable journey of pregnancy and motherhood ahead.

Changes during the First Trimester

I will state this repeatedly in this book so apologies in advance; every pregnancy is different. On this basis, the symptoms here are not a definitive guide of what to expect. However if you are aware of them and appropriate self-care techniques, it can make your pregnancy more empowering and enjoyable.

Common 1st Trimester symptoms include:

- Morning sickness or nausea
- Heartburn or acid reflux
- Headaches or migraines
- Lower back or pelvic pain
- Tender swollen breasts
- Constipation.
- Polyuria
- Cravings

Hormones

Relaxin is a hormone produced by the corpus luteum of the ovaries and the decidua of the placenta. It is named as such for its role in relaxing joint tissues in later stages of pregnancy. In the first trimester, relaxin peaks in concentration and is thought to be involved with placental implantation and growth (Bermas, B., et al 2017). This peak, along with the anterior tilt of the pelvis, can cause discomfort to the lower back and pelvic region in the first trimester.

During pregnancy **oestrogen** levels can rise up to 100 times the amount found in women who are not pregnant (Novakovic, A. 2017). In the first trimester the amount of oestrogen rises sharply as the placenta takes over as the primary source of production. This increase is considered to be one of the causes of morning sickness, is responsible for maintaining the growth of the uterus as well as suppression of hormones that cause ovulation (Brighten, J. 2021).

Progesterone hormone levels also increase. This relaxes muscles in the uterus to allow its expansion and prevent early childbirth. This can also relax the muscles in the stomach and intestine walls, resulting in excess stomach acids and acid reflux (Novakovic, A. 2017).

Human chorionic gonadotropin (hCG) is first produced by the developing embryo soon after conception, then later by the placenta. This hormone is detected by pregnancy tests as is present in your urine or blood a few days after implantation. Typically, concentrations of hCG rise exponentially in the first trimester of pregnancy, doubling about every 24 hours during the first 8 weeks (Betz, D. et al 2023). Some experts suggest there may be a link between hCG levels and morning sickness. Higher hCG levels have been found in women with morning sickness compared to those who are asymptomatic (Masson, G., et al. 1985). Furthermore in a 1992 study hCG levels correlated positively with the severity of nausea and vomiting in women with hyperemesis gravidarum

Cavity Pressure Changes

Once an egg is fertilised, it takes about 7 days to attach to the lining of the uterus. This lining, known as the endometrium, becomes thicker to provide nutrients to the developing embryo. The uterus changes shape to allow room for the embryo. This can cause mild cramping. The endometrium continues to thicken and the uterus gradually expands as the embryo grows. The growing uterus mass causes an increase in pressure on other organs in the lower pelvic cavity. As a result you may experience an increase in urination from increased cavity pressure on the bladder and towards the end of the trimester you may also become constipated. It is believed hormones are also involved in the changes to pelvic organ functions.

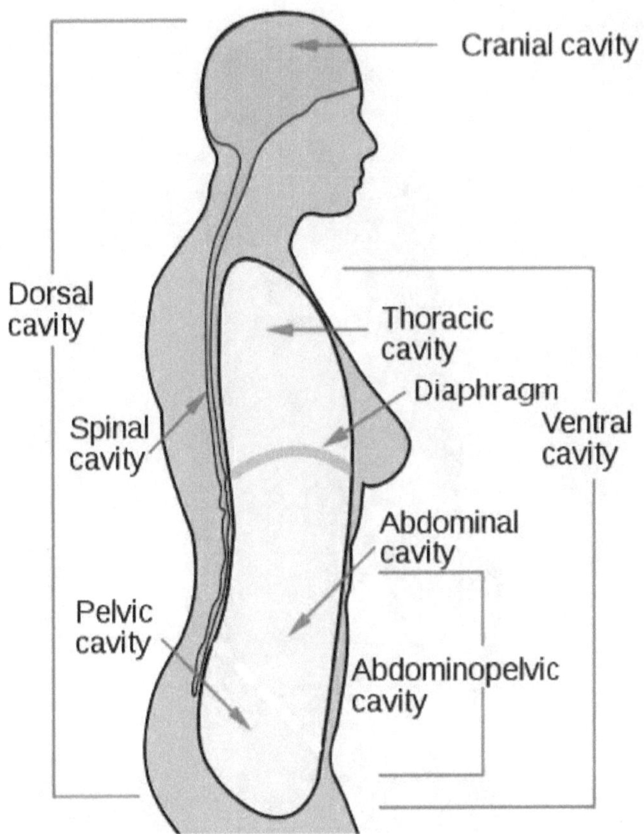

Musculoskeletal Changes

As the embryo grows the uterus expands outwards as well as up. Adapting to the pressure changes and increased weight, the pelvis begins to tilt anteriorly. This tilt increases the rear facing curve (lordosis) of the lower back. By week 12 the lower back curve can increase in by up to 6.7°(Rahimi, A. Et al 2015). These changes to the pelvis and lower spine alter tissue tensions and pressure which can cause discomfort and lower back pain.

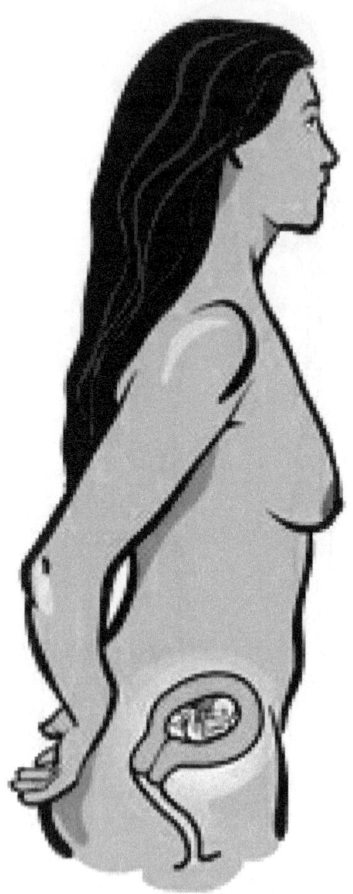

It is common for breasts to become tender and swell during the first trimester. For some they may also grow in size. This adds weight to the front of the rib cage and can create tension in the shoulders and upper back. In addition to this, both the breast weight and pelvic tilt can cause the shoulders to roll forward increasing the forward curve (kyphosis) of the upper back. By week 12 the upper back curve can increase by up to 5.4° (Rahimi, A. Et al 2015). This can result in anterior head carriage, creating tension through the neck muscles and headaches.

Morning Sickness

The first trimester is often met with morning sickness. Morning sickness is easily the most common disorder in pregnancy. Most experience nausea or vomiting in the morning, hence the name, but the severity and time scale vary; the most severe form is known as hyperemesis gravidarum. Morning sickness can begin as early as two weeks in to the pregnancy. There is still no full understanding of why this occurs but there is belief that hormones produced by the placenta may be an affecting factor. There are also possible links between morning sickness and low blood sugar levels (hypoglycaemia) in the first trimester (Novakovic, A. 2017).

Scents have been known to trigger nausea and vomiting in pregnancy due to heightened senses. Hyperosmia is an increased sensitivity to smells that can occur during pregnancy. The cause of this is not understood, but as with most pregnancy symptoms, it is thought to be a result of hormone changes. Your perception of certain smells can also change, from smelling perfumes walking past a shop to a whiff of fresh coffee turning your stomach. There are discussions about hyperosmia providing a protective function against toxin ingestion however this lacks research so remains a theory until more studies are done.

For years it has been claimed that morning sickness prevents pregnancy loss but this was only confirmed in 2016, when researchers did a second reading of a study on aspirin as a potential preventative. In a randomised trial, pregnant women with previous losses were studied to observe live births and pregnancy losses with or without aspirin. While there was no noticeable effect with that study, the team analysed the participants' journal data and discovered a inverse link between morning sickness and pregnancy loss with the hazard rate for all types of loss being less than half of the rate for those without morning sickness (Hinkle et al, 2016).

There are various suggested methods to relieve morning sickness including:

- Eating dry toast or a dry biscuit (like rich tea) before you get out of bed.

- Eating small (non-greasy) meals often.
- Eating cold foods instead of hot ones.
- Ginger foods or drinks have been shown to reduce nausea and vomiting. Ginger biscuits worked for me!
- Acupuncture or acupressure is shown to help with morning sickness and is also shown to be more effective for hyperemesis gravidarum than conventional methods (Lu et al, 2021).
- Osteopathy can help with symptoms related to morning sickness and hyperemesis gravidarum such as mid back pain, diaphragm muscle balancing and jaw muscle relaxation.

Every body is different and while one might work for someone, two or more may be better for someone else. It is advisable to get plenty of rest and stay hydrated by frequently sipping water. Water can help reduce vomiting by diluting the stomach acids.

Exercise To Help With Morning Sickness Or Hyperemesis Gravidarum

Smile Stretch

This exercise can be done seated or laying down.
Smile as widely as you can comfortably.
While smiling, lower your jaw 2 inches.
Inhale and as you exhale slowly relax your smile and bring your jaw back up.
Repeat 3 times.
Perform once a day.

This exercise loosens jaw muscles which can become sore from morning sickness.

Acid Reflux

Gastroesophageal reflux disease (GERD) is reported in up to 80% of pregnancies. The most common symptoms of GERD are acid reflux and resulting heartburn (Law et al, 2010). In some studies, the prevalence of heartburn has been found to increase from 22% in the first trimester to 39% in the second trimester to between 60% and 72% in the third trimester. However, one prospective cohort study found that, in most pregnant women, heartburn, acid regurgitation, or both began in the first trimester and disappeared during the second trimester (Vazquez, 2015). Increased progesterone levels and changes in body cavity pressure can cause acid reflux as early as the first trimester. Hormonal changes in pregnancy can also decrease gastric motility, resulting in prolonged gastric emptying time and increased risk of reflux (Law et al 2010). Upper chest breathing from stress and altered abdominal pressure can also reduce diaphragm use. Studies conducted during the last 10 years show that there are two lower oesophageal muscular rings, known as sphincters, which are partially made from diaphragm tissue. (Mittal, R., 1998). This suggests the reduced use of the diaphragm can also weaken the sphincters between the oesophagus and the stomach. This weakness allows stomach acids to move in to the oesophagus, causing heartburn.

Methods to manage GERD symptoms include:

- Eating smaller meals more frequently,
- Consuming ginger products, such as ginger biscuits or tea
- Avoiding fatty or acidic foods
- Avoid eating near bedtime
- Elevating the head of the bed
- Using antacid medications such as Gaviscon

Exercise To Prevent Or Reduce Acid Reflux

Diaphragmatic Breathing

Lie flat on the floor, your bed, or another comfortable, flat surface.
Put a hand on your chest and a hand on your stomach.
Breathe in through your nose. During this type of breathing, make sure your stomach is expanding while your chest remains relatively still.
press gently on your stomach, and exhale slowly feeling your stomach contract as your breathe out.

- Repeat 10 times.
- Perform once a day.

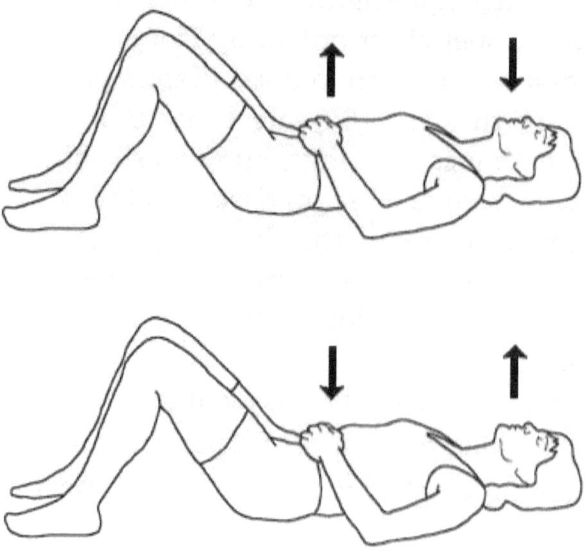

This exercise can help improve the tone of your diaphragm and in turn reduce the laxity of the lower oesophageal sphincters, helping reduce or prevent acid reflux as well as morning sickness.

Headaches And Migraines

In the first trimester, hormones, decreased blood sugar levels, posture and even hyperosmia can contribute to headaches and migraines.

Anterior head carriage from rolled shoulders can also pull the posterior neck muscles, resulting in tension headaches. Around 26% of pregnancy headaches are tension headaches.

Pregnancy will usually reduce the frequency and severity of migraine attacks. Migraine attacks often increase in frequency in the first trimester but can be expected to decrease later in pregnancy. However, although attacks are usually less frequent in the second and third trimesters, new onset aura may appear at that time (Goadsby et al, 2008). Migraines are often triggered by certain food types so it is advisable to avoid these where possible if you suffer with migraines prior to pregnancy.

Other causes of headaches include:

- Dehydration
- Nausea and vomiting
- Stress
- Poor nutrition
- Caffeine withdrawal
- Lack of sleep
- Certain foods

The majority of headache causes are treatable through self care! Reading this book is the first step, but taking action gets results. If there was ever a time to take care of yourself, during pregnancy would be one of the most important.

Exercises To Relieve Headaches

Supine Chin Tuck

While lying on your back with a small pillow or towel under your head, tuck your chin towards your chest. Maintain contact of your head with the surface you are lying on the entire time.

- Hold for 20 Seconds
- Repeat twice
- Perform once a Day

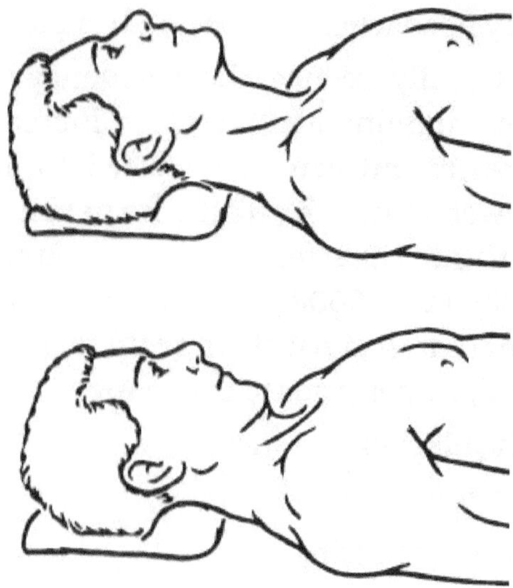

This exercise helps rebalance the position of your head and neck by working muscles at the front of your neck and gently stretching muscles at the base of the skull and the back of the neck.

Seated Neck Stretch

While sitting in a chair, hook one hand under the seat of the chair. Lift your other arm over the side of your head and gently direct your head and neck away from the opposite side.

Do the same using opposite hands and directions to stretch the other side.

- Hold for 20 seconds
- Repeat once each side.
- Perform once a day.

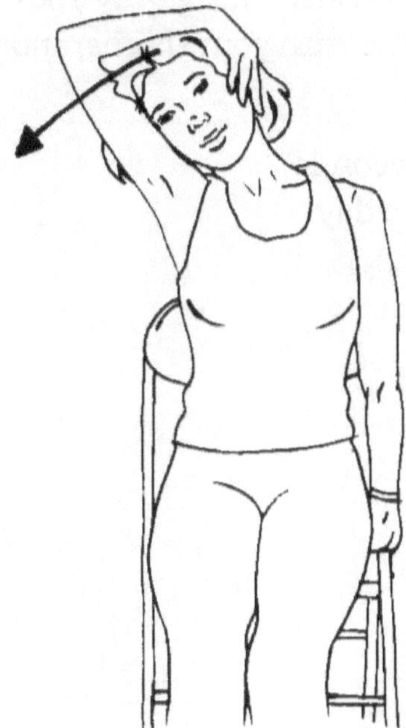

This stretch focuses on the side muscles of your neck which can shorten when your shoulders and head are held in a forward position. Stretching these can help reduce neck compression as well as improving the blood flow to and from your head.

Lower Back Or Pelvic Pain

To accommodate the growing baby, anterior pelvic tilt and the resulting lower back compression can cause lower back and pelvic pain in the first trimester.

Constipation can also contribute to lower back pain. Eating foods rich in fibre and drinking warm water can help to relieve this.

Exercises To Relieve Lower Back Pain

Pelvic Tilt

Lay on your back with your knees bent and feet placed firmly on the floor (or mattress if choosing to do this in bed). Take a deep breath in, and as you breathe out gently rock your pelvis to lift your tail bone up - in line with your thighs, and press your tummy in to the floor.

- Hold for 20 seconds
- Repeat twice a day

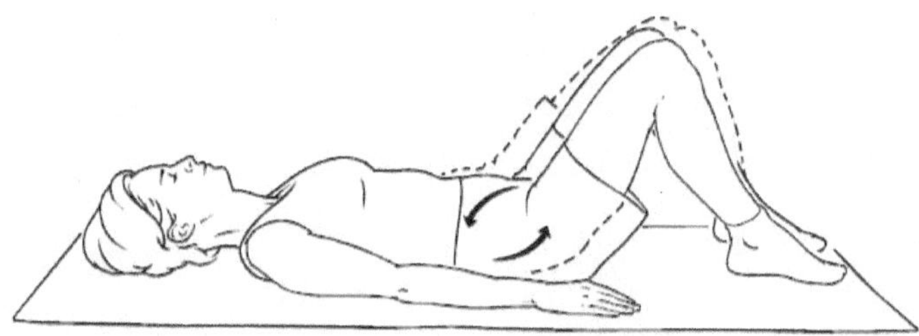

This exercise helps to mobilise your lower back, engage your core muscles and hip extensor muscles.

Nutrition

I found during pregnancy women are bombarded with information about foods to avoid and remove from their diets. This can be disheartening, especially for those who love shellfish.

So to counter the restrictive lists I have made inclusive lists of nutrients to support pregnancy as well as lists of food with an approximate amount of the nutrient per 100g of the food item.

These lists can help you formulate a diet you can enjoy while nuturing your body's needs.

Folate

Folate (vitamin B9), together with vitamin B12, is required to form red blood cells. A deficiency in folate can reduce the ability of red blood cells to carry oxygen, this is called "macrocytic" anaemia. It is also essential for DNA replication, protein (amino acid) synthesis and vitamin metabolism (Greenberg et al, 2011).

In the first few weeks of pregnancy, the foetus rapidly develops spine and nerve cells. During this time, folate plays a significant role in the baby's spine. Supplementation of this vitamin helps to prevent the development of a 'neural tube defect', resulting in a spinal malformation called spina bifida.

Folic acid is the term used for the synthetic dietary supplement used to enrich foods and vitamin supplements.

According to the British Dietetic Association:

While conceiving the recommended daily intake is 200µg of folic acid plus a supplement* containing 400µg.

During pregnancy a daily intake is 300µg of folic acid plus a 400µg supplement* during the first 12 weeks of pregnancy.

* You may need to take 5mg/d of folic acid preconception and up to 12 weeks of pregnancy i.e. if you have had a pregnancy previously affected by neural tube defects or if you have diabetes or take anti-epilepsy medication

Foods containing high amounts of folate:

Edamame (green soybeans) - 311μg per 100g.

Lentils - 181μg per 100g.

Asparagus -149μg per 100g

Spinach - 146μg per 100g

Broccoli - 108μg per 100g

Avocado - 81μg per 100g

Iron is used by your body to make haemoglobin, a protein in the red blood cells that carries oxygen to your tissues. During pregnancy, your body needs double the amount of iron to supply oxygen to the developing foetus.

Having adequate iron levels can prevent a condition called iron deficiency anaemia. This condition is known to cause tiredness and severe headaches. Anaemia can also affect premature labour and development of the baby.

According to WebMD:

During pregnancy a minimum iron intake of 27mg is recommended daily.

Breastfeeding mothers are recommended a minimum iron intake of 9mg daily.

Foods containing high amounts of iron:

Baking Chocolate - 17.4mg per 100g

Squash or pumpkin seeds - 8.8mg per 100g

Lean Beef - 5.5mg per 100g

Edamame (green soybeans) - 5.1mg per 100g

Spinach - 3.6mg per 100g

Lentils - 3.3mg per 100g

Calcium

Calcium is essential for foetal bone development, as well as muscle, heart and nerve development. Regardless of how much calcium you consume, your body will take what is needed for the developing foetus.

According to WebMD:

> During pregnancy a minimum calcium intake of 1000mg is recommended daily.*

> The same is recommended for breastfeeding mothers.*

*If under 19 years old 1300mg daily intake is recommended.

Foods containing high amounts of calcium:

Cheddar cheese - 710mg per 100g

Kale - 254mg per 100g

Garlic - 181mg per 100g

Edamame (green soybeans) - 145mg per 100g

Spinach - 136mg per 100g

Whole milk - 113mg per 100g

Part Two

The Second Trimester

The Second Trimester

> *"Let us make pregnancy an occasion
> when we appreciate our female bodies."*

– Merete Leonhardt-Lupa

Every person's pregnancy experience is different, in fact every pregnancy is varied overall, but there are some consistencies that the majority of women experience. Morning sickness can start to subside by the second trimester and cravings can start to form. The bladder may seem less persistent than before and for some women the little bump will be starting to show.

The second trimester is often seen as a safety milestone in pregnancy. This means you can begin looking at antenatal activities as well as knowing certain (carefully applied) manual treatments can be applied for any physocal ailments that need attention.

NB: please ensure you reserach any practitioners in relation to pregnancy treatments prior before booking.

Antenatal Activities

Over the past decade there has been an increase in antenatal services helping both parents prepare for the arrival of their baby, meaning families are no longer limited to antenatal classes.

Sampling different techniques allows you to cherry pick what feels comfortable, giving you a better understanding of your options. This allows you to make informed choices to prepare for pregnancy changes, labour and recovery. Attending various groups and classes also allows you to meet other expecting parents. This can help you by giving you people in a similar situation to talk to as well as increasing your social support network throughout your pregnancy, often found to be an unexpected blessing!

Please note:

If you have any of the following conditions consult your doctor or midwife before undertaking any form of antenatal exercise classes:

- PIH (Pregnancy Induced Hypertension)
- Pre-eclampsia
- Cardiac disease
- IUGR (Intra Uterine Growth Retardation)
- A history of two or more miscarriages
- A history of premature labour
- Unexplained vaginal bleeding
- Placenta praevia (a low-lying placenta)

Antenatal Classes

As you are now in the second trimester it is a perfect time to start finding out about local antenatal classes.

Antenatal classes start around 30 weeks but can be accessed

earlier in special cases or if private. They offer numerous benefits for expectant parents as they prepare for childbirth and parenthood. Firstly, these classes provide essential education about pregnancy, labour, and childbirth, helping parents understand the physical and emotional changes they can expect during this time. They also teach practical skills such as breathing techniques, relaxation methods, and positions for labour and birth, which can help reduce anxiety and increase confidence during labour. Additionally, antenatal classes often cover topics related to newborn care, breastfeeding, and post-partum recovery, equipping parents with valuable knowledge to care for their baby and themselves after childbirth. Participating in these classes also offers an opportunity for expectant parents to connect with others going through similar experiences, building a support network that can extend beyond the classroom. Classes are available on the NHS but it is worth joining local online forums to discuss with other mums about which are good to use, private classes are used more now than NHS ones as a result of poor experiences, the more you know the easier it is to make an informed choice!

Acupuncture

Acupuncture, a cornerstone of traditional Chinese medicine (TCM) dating back thousands of years, has garnered global recognition for its holistic approach to health and wellness. Rooted in the concept of Qi (pronounced "chee"), the vital life force that flows through pathways or meridians in the body, acupuncture aims to restore balance and harmony to these energy channels. Through the strategic insertion of thin needles into specific points along these meridians, acupuncturists seek to alleviate a myriad of ailments, ranging from chronic pain and musculoskeletal disorders to stress, anxiety, and digestive issues. Despite its ancient origins, acupuncture continues to evolve, integrating modern scientific research to validate its efficacy and mechanisms of action.

Contemporary studies suggest that acupuncture stimulates the release of endorphins and neurotransmitters, such as serotonin and dopamine, which contribute to pain relief and mood regulation. Furthermore, acupuncture's ability to modulate the autonomic nervous system and regulate inflammatory responses has broadened its applications in complementary and alternative medicine.Acupuncture can be used alongside other forms of therapy to help reduce painful symptoms of pregnancy as well as to help prepare the body for labour.

Benefits of Acupuncture:
- Reducing musculoskeletal pain
- Easing symptoms of hyperemesis
- Improved mental well-being
- Improved energy levels
- Softens the cervix in preparation for labour

Antenatal Yoga

If you are an active person and would like to remain so during pregnancy, antenatal yoga is one option to do just that. Antenatal yoga, also known as prenatal yoga, has emerged as a popular practice for expectant mothers seeking to nurture their physical, mental, and emotional well-being throughout pregnancy. Rooted in the ancient tradition of yoga, antenatal yoga classes are specifically tailored to accommodate the changing needs and limitations of pregnant women. These classes typically incorporate gentle yoga postures, breathing exercises, meditation, and relaxation techniques, all designed to support the mother's journey through pregnancy, labor, and childbirth. Through mindful movement and breathwork, antenatal yoga aims to alleviate common discomforts associated with pregnancy, such as back pain, sciatica, and swelling, while also promoting strength, flexibility, and balance. Moreover, the emphasis on deep breathing and relaxation techniques helps expecting mothers cultivate a sense of calm, reduce stress and anxiety, and enhance their connection with their baby. Beyond the physical benefits, antenatal yoga classes provide a supportive community where mothers-to-be can share experiences, fears, and joys, fostering a sense of belonging and empowerment during this transformative time. With its focus on holistic wellness and empowerment, antenatal yoga offers pregnant women a nurturing space to embrace the journey of motherhood with grace, mindfulness, and self-compassion.

Antenatal yoga is adapted to prevent straining the abdominal muscles and considers the changes to your musculoskeletal system, including the relaxation of tissues caused by the hormone relaxin.

Antenatal yoga classes are gentle and flowing but each one can be tailored to your needs as there are less attendees than regular classes to allow the teacher to be more attemtive. The classes can be started during the second trimester and continued throughout, helping reduce and prevent pregnancy related issues such as back pain and swollen ankles.

Benefits of Antenatal Yoga:
- Encourages mind and body connection
- Teaches breathing techniques to aid relaxation throughout pregnancy and labour
- Improves sleep
- Supports the body during postural changes
- Provides relief from common pregnancy complaints
- Promotes connection with your baby
- Helps you to make friends with other expecting families

Aquanatal

AquaNatal classes, also referred to as prenatal aqua aerobics or water-based prenatal exercise, offer expectant mothers a unique and effective way to stay fit and healthy during the second and third trimester. These classes, typically conducted in a pool setting, cater specifically to the needs of pregnant women, providing a safe and supportive environment for gentle yet effective workouts. The buoyancy of water alleviates the strain on the joints and ligaments, making it an ideal exercise option for relieving common discomforts such as back pain, swelling, and pressure on the pelvis. AquaNatal exercises often incorporate a combination of cardiovascular, strength, and flexibility training, utilizing the resistance of water to enhance muscle tone and endurance while improving circulation and reducing fluid retention. Moreover, the supportive atmosphere of AquaNatal classes fosters a sense of camaraderie among expectant mothers, allowing them to connect, share experiences, and build a supportive community. Beyond the physical benefits, participating in AquaNatal classes can also promote relaxation, stress reduction, and emotional well-being, as the soothing properties of water provide a calming effect on both the body and mind. Overall, AquaNatal classes offer pregnant women a holistic approach to prenatal fitness, helping them stay active, healthy, and prepared for the journey of childbirth and motherhood.

You do not have to be able to swim to do this class as you are in a comfortable depth of water to allow you to fele feel safe while exercising. Floats can also be provided if required.

Benefits of AquaNatal:
- Improves sleep
- Improves circulation
- Reduces fluid retention

- Improves balance and coordination
- Maintenance of cardiovascular fitness

Hypnobirthing

Hypnobirthing empowers expectant mothers with techniques to achieve a calm, relaxed, and positive birthing experience. Rooted in the belief that fear and tension can exacerbate pain during labor, hypnobirthing teaches women how to enter a state of deep relaxation through self-hypnosis, visualization, breathing techniques, and affirmations. By practicing these techniques throughout pregnancy, mothers-to-be learn to trust their bodies' innate ability to birth their babies naturally and without unnecessary medical interventions. Hypnobirthing emphasizes the role of the mind-body connection in childbirth, encouraging women to release fears and anxieties surrounding labor and replace them with confidence and trust. Additionally, partners are actively involved in the process, learning how to support and advocate for the birthing mother while creating a peaceful and supportive birthing environment. The benefits of hypnobirthing extend beyond the birthing experience itself, with many participants reporting reduced pain, shorter labor durations, and a greater sense of empowerment and satisfaction with their birthing experiences. As hypnobirthing continues to gain recognition, it offers expectant parents a holistic and empowering approach to childbirth, promoting a positive and transformative journey into parenthood.

HypnoBirthing is beneficial for mothers who have previously experienced traumatic labours.

While the techniques used in HypnoBirthing cannot prevent unforeseeable complications they can have a positive impact on the way that you respond to them.

Benefits of HypnoBirthing:

- Managing stress hormones throughout pregnancy and

labour
- Giving the mother the feeling of control
- Reducing the need for pain relieving drugs
- Reducing the need for medical intervention
- Improving the speed of delivery and overall experience of childbirth

Pregnancy Pilates

Pregnancy Pilates is a specialized form of exercise tailored to the unique needs and physical changes experienced by expectant mothers. It combines elements of traditional Pilates with modifications that accommodate the various stages of pregnancy, focusing on strengthening the core muscles, improving flexibility, and enhancing overall body awareness. One of the key benefits of Pregnancy Pilates is its emphasis on pelvic floor health, which is crucial during pregnancy and childbirth. By engaging in controlled movements and exercises, pregnant women can strengthen their pelvic floor muscles, which can help alleviate common discomforts such as back pain and pelvic instability. Additionally, Pregnancy Pilates can aid in maintaining proper posture and alignment as the body undergoes significant changes, helping to reduce strain on the spine and joints. Moreover, the breathing techniques incorporated into Pregnancy Pilates sessions promote relaxation and stress reduction, which can be particularly beneficial during pregnancy. It's essential to note that Pregnancy Pilates should be practiced under the guidance of a certified instructor who has experience working with pregnant women to ensure safety and effectiveness. Overall, Pregnancy Pilates offers a gentle yet effective way for expectant mothers to stay active, alleviate discomfort, and prepare their bodies for the demands of childbirth.

Pregnancy Pilates exercises are focused on the abdominals, back and pelvic floor muscles to reduce pregnancy related pains and help with postnatal recovery.

Benefits of Pregnancy Pilates:

- Improved core strength
- Improved pregnancy posture
- Prevention and relief from common pregnancy complaints
- Improved pelvic floor strength
- Better stability and coordination
- Improves postnatal recovery
- As with antenatal yoga, it helps you meet other expecting families

Birth Plan

Now that you are in the second trimester it is worth thinking about what you would like to happen during your labour.

During pregnancy, expectant parents often find themselves navigating a multitude of decisions, from choosing healthcare providers to making preparations for childbirth. Amidst these considerations, the birth plan emerges as a vital tool for expecting families, serving as a roadmap that outlines their preferences and wishes for labour and delivery. While some may perceive it as a rigid script, a birth plan is, in essence, a communication tool that fosters collaboration and empowerment between parents-to-be and their healthcare team.

At its core, a birth plan provides an opportunity for expectant parents to articulate their preferences regarding various aspects of labour, delivery, and postpartum care (see Part Four: The Fourth Trimester). These preferences may range from pain management options to the ambiance of the birthing environment, from preferences for medical interventions to desires for immediate skin-to-skin contact with the newborn. By documenting these preferences in a birth plan, parents can ensure that their voices are heard and respected throughout the childbirth process.

Moreover, the process of creating a birth plan encourages expectant parents to educate themselves about the various options and possibilities surrounding childbirth. Researching topics such as different birthing positions, pain relief methods, and potential interventions empowers parents to make informed decisions that align with their values and preferences. In this sense, the birth plan becomes not only a document but also a tool for self-advocacy and informed choice.

Importantly, a birth plan serves as a catalyst for communication and collaboration between expectant parents and their healthcare providers. By discussing the contents of the birth plan with their obstetrician, midwife, or doula, parents can ensure that their preferences are understood and feasible within the context of their medical situation. This dialogue fosters a sense of partnership and mutual understanding, laying the foundation for a positive birthing experience characterised by trust and respect.

Furthermore, a birth plan can help mitigate anxiety and uncertainty surrounding childbirth by providing a sense of structure and predictability. By envisioning and documenting their ideal birth scenario, parents-to-be can cultivate a sense of agency and control in an otherwise unpredictable process. While childbirth is inherently unpredictable and plans may need to adapt in response to unforeseen circumstances, having a birth plan in place can instill a sense of preparedness and confidence in expectant parents.

In addition to outlining preferences for labour and delivery, a birth plan can also encompass postpartum wishes and intentions. From preferences for breastfeeding support to plans for newborn care and bonding, the birth plan extends beyond the moment of birth to encompass the early postpartum period. By addressing these considerations proactively, parents can set the stage for a smoother transition into parenthood and optimize the support available to them during this critical period.

Birth plans play a crucial role in the childbirth journey, serving as a means of expressing preferences, fostering communication, and promoting informed decision-making. While childbirth is inherently unpredictable, a birth plan empowers expectant parents to advocate for their needs and desires, collaborate with their healthcare team, and navigate the complexities of childbirth with confidence and clarity. As a tool for empowerment and self-advocacy, the birth plan holds immense value in shaping a positive and fulfilling birthing experience for expectant families.

Association for Improvements in the Maternity Services

The Association for Improvements in the Maternity Services (AiMS) is a trusted source of information on what you can request in your birth plan depending on your personal circumstances.

Informing yourself ahead of a conversation with your midwife will help you feel more prepared and empowered. Their website is included in the links section.

What should be included?
You may wish to include things like:

- Your birthing partner
- The venue you would like to give birth
- Pain relief to use or avoid
- Positions you would like to try while in labour
- Special facilities (such as a birthing pool)
- Special requirements such as a translator or sign language interpreter
- Delayed cord clamping preferences.
- Skin to skin time after the birth
- Whether you are planning to breastfeed so you are supported with the first few feeds.

Once written it is good to share your birth plan with both your birth partner and midwife so they aware of your choices.

Changes during the Second Trimester

The second trimester of pregnancy, often considered the golden period, typically spans from weeks 13 to 28 and brings about a multitude of changes and milestones for expectant mothers. Physically, many women find relief from the discomforts of the first trimester, such as nausea and fatigue, as energy levels increase and the infamous "pregnancy glow" may make its appearance. During this time, the uterus expands significantly, causing the baby bump to become more pronounced and often leading to a heightened sense of awareness of the growing life within. For many expectant parents, the second trimester marks the eagerly anticipated milestone of feeling the baby's first movements, known as "quickening," which can foster a deeper connection with the developing fetus. Additionally, prenatal appointments become more frequent during the second trimester, allowing healthcare providers to monitor fetal growth and development closely, conduct routine screenings, and provide expectant parents with valuable information and support. Emotionally, the second trimester may bring a sense of excitement and anticipation as the reality of impending parenthood becomes more tangible. Couples often begin to bond more deeply with their unborn child, engaging in activities such as shopping for baby essentials, attending prenatal classes, and even choosing a name. While the second trimester is generally characterized by increased energy and a sense of well-being, it's important to acknowledge that every pregnancy is unique, and expectant mothers may still encounter challenges such as back pain, heartburn, and mood swings. Overall, the second trimester represents a period of growth, anticipation, and preparation as expectant parents eagerly await the arrival of their bundle of joy. Morning sickness tends to lessen by this time as does the fatigue and breast tenderness. These changes are due to a decrease in levels of human chorionic gonadotropin (hCG) hormone and an adjustment to the levels of oestrogen and progesterone hormones.

Common 2nd trimester symptoms:

- Cravings.
- Mood swings.
- Feeling the first movement of the baby (quickening)
- Pain around the sides of the lower abdomen
- Headaches (see 1st trimester)
- Heartburn/acid reflux (see 1st trimester)
- Bloating and constipation.
- Sore breasts.
- Shoulder pains
- Leg cramps.
- Swollen feet.
- Stiffness in lower back

Cravings

Some women experience cravings before they even know they are pregnant (mine was sprouts about a week before I knew!). Cravings are normal despite how bizarre they may be and can often be a result of your body telling you it needs something!

You may also find that certain foods you used to like make you feel nauseous, as well as certain smells. This is all the result of the change in your microbiome (gut bacteria), hormones and immune system while your body prioritises the growth and protection of your baby.

It can be amusing discussing these changes with other expecting families, as every body has a unique response.

Mood Swings

Your body is undergoing significant changes, both physically and hormonally, to accommodate the growing baby. These changes can also have an effect on the manner in which you react to your circumstances. By week 20 women can often begin a process called "nesting". This is where you find yourself reorganising or fixing issues in the household, it can also be displayed as a lower tolerance to things you had previously accepted, such as bad habits, messiness and so on. The latter nesting symptoms are often called mood swings but are in my opinion a natural part of the nesting process, creating a comfortable and safe environment for yourself and the baby.

Sometimes we can allow these changes to affect us in a negative way, causing antenatal anxiety or depression. It is worth speaking with your midwife if you find that you are becoming overwhelmed emotionally and they can advise on helpful steps to take.

Quickening

Between weeks 17 and 20 you may feel a fluttering sensation in your lower abdomen. This is the first time you are feeling your baby move and is called quickening. From this point onwards you will become more aware of your baby's movements, especially later at night when you settle to sleep!

Hormones

Hormones are still changing in the 2nd trimester but much less so than in the first.

Oestrogen and **progesterone** continue to increase to support the baby's growth. These hormones also stimulate the **melanocyte-stimulating hormone.** Melanocyte cells produce melanin which has a variety of biological functions, including skin and hair pigmentation and photo-protection of the skin and eyes (Schlessinger, D., et al 2021). This can result in melasma (brown or greyish patches on the face), linea nigra (the dark line in the centre of the lower abdomen) as well as the darkening of the areolae around the nipples.

Cortisol is a stress hormone which has been mentioned in the first trimester. However, this hormone is not limited to stress reactions and is necessary during pregnancy to regulate your metabolism and control blood sugar levels. High levels of cortisol are associated with symptoms like stretch marks, blood pressure issues, and added redness in the face.

Human placental lactogen (HPL) is a hormone secreted from the placenta and is thought to help the baby grow. It's also one of the main hormones associated with insulin resistance during pregnancy, or gestational diabetes, as it can increase the mother's blood sugar levels by having a blocking effect on insulin.

Cavity Pressure Changes

The uterus continues to expand making room for the baby, This puts pressure on nearby muscles and ligaments and can cause cramps in your lower abdomen and back. The uterus begins to grow upward and out of the pelvic cavity, reducing pressure on the bladder. This pressure change can cause the rib cage to lift upward to accommodate the expanding uterus (Stone, C., 2007). If the rib cage doesn't lift, pressure on the abdominal organs and the diaphragm muscle will increase. This can lead to constipation, acid reflux (heartburn) and shortness of breath.

Musculoskeletal Changes

The growing baby and breasts continue to affect the mother's centre of mass and weight distribution. This causes continuous postural changes which are then counter balanced with compensatory changes throughout the spine.

The pelvis can tilt further forward by up to 6.3°, causing the lumbar spine to curve up to 7.3° more (Kouhkan, S., et al 2015). This curve with the increasing anterior weight in the abdominal cavity can cause lower back discomfort and some cases sciatica as a result of narrowing intervertebral space causing nerve irritation.

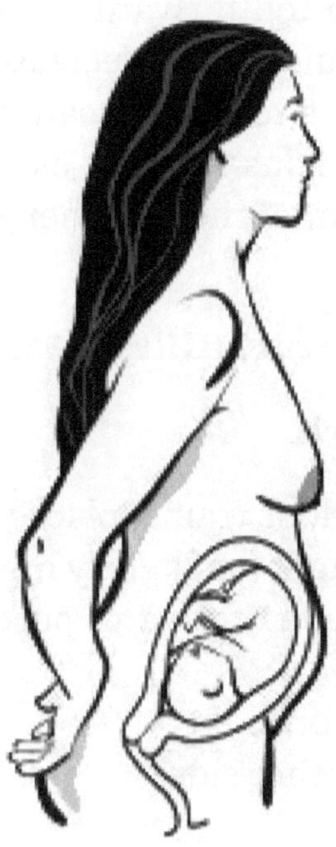

There is also an increase in hip external rotation which correlates with a larger step width (Mei, Q., et al 2018). This can also contribute to sciatica nerve irritation due to shortening of the piriformis muscle in relation to the hips external rotation. Pronation of the feet can also increase during the second trimester, increasing pressure through the inner arch of the foot and potentially reducing plantar flexion of the ankle (Conder, R., et al 2019). This can result in plantar fasciitis pain as well as swollen ankles, ankle stiffness and leg cramps.

The additional weight of the growing breasts can also cause the mother's shoulders to roll forward, increasing tension through the upper trapezius muscles. This can result in shoulder pains as well as tension headaches.

Shoulder Pains

As the breasts develop and increase in size the added weight can cause your shoulders to roll forward. This increases the tension through your upper shoulders and decreases the space at the front of the shoulder joint. As a result you can experience tension pain through the upper trapezius muscles as well as pinching of the biceps tendon at the front of the shoulder joint.

Exercise To Relieve Shoulder Pain.

Standing Pectoral stretch.

- Standing in a door frame, place you forearm and elbow at shoulder height (or slightly higher) on the door frame
- Walk the same leg forward, putting your weight on to the front leg.
- Hold for 20 seconds
- Repeat on the other side

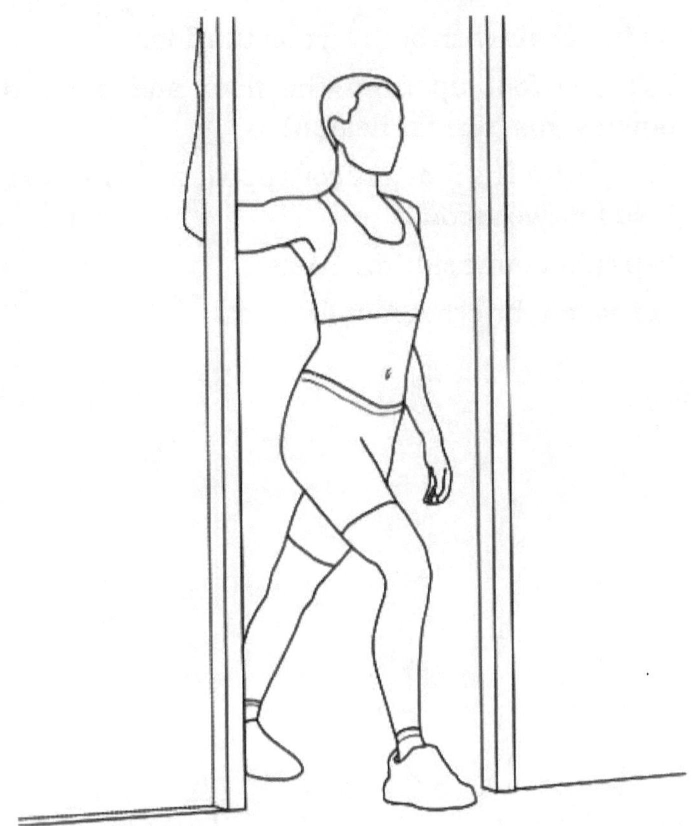

This exercise stretches your pectoral muscles and helps you open up your chest, reducing pressure on the front shoulder joint and reducing tension through your upper trapezius muscles.

Leg Cramps

Due to the change in weight distribution and relaxation of ligaments throughout the body, the use of lower leg muscles adapts in response to these changes and can result in leg cramps, stiffness and swelling of the feet.

Gentle exercises such as walking or swimming can help prevent leg cramps and swelling.

Exercises to prevent leg cramps

Ankle Flexing

- Sit in a chair with both feet on the floor
- Lift one foot up from the floor and point the toes downwards (plantar flexion)
- Then point the foot and toes upwards (dorsiflexion) and hold for two seconds
- Repeat on same side for 5 sets
- Repeat on the other foot for 5 sets

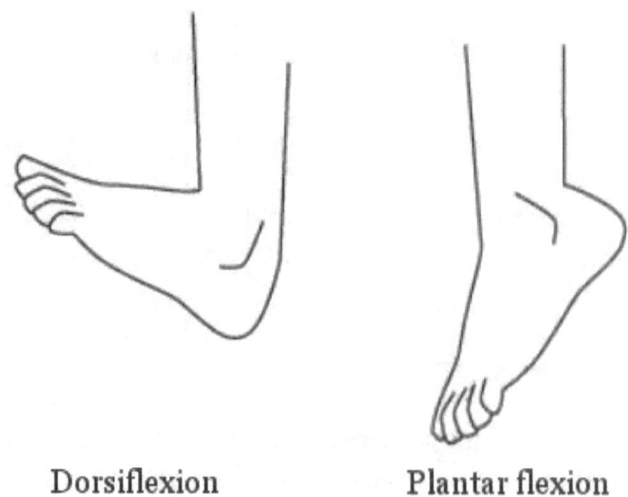

Dorsiflexion   Plantar flexion

This exercise helps to mobilise the ankle, stretches the calf and shin muscles gently as well as helping to pump fluids away from the foot and ankle.

Ankle rotations

- Stay seated as with the previous exercise.
- Lift one leg up and rotate the foot and toes in a clockwise motion 5 times.
- Repeat in an anti clockwise direction.
- Repeat on opposite leg in both directions.

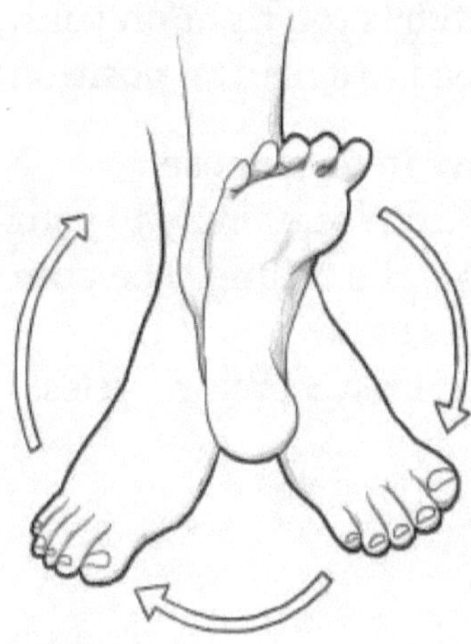

This exercise helps mobilise the ankle while both strengthening and stretching muscles in the lower leg.

Back Stiffness

As the baby and breasts develop, weight is added to the front of the body causing the spine to adapt to the added load. This can result in the spine becoming stiff and sore, especially in the lumbar (lower) area. The lumbar spine can arch further, narrowing the posterior spine and potentially leading to nerve irritation or sciatica.

Exercise for back stiffness.

Cat/Cow pose.

- Come on to your hands and knees with your hands below the shoulders, and knees below the hips.
- Begin by moving in to cow pose.
- Inhale and lower your belly towards the floor or mat.

- Lift your chin and chest, and gaze up toward the ceiling (if this stretch is too tight on your abdomen, lower your chin and head to a neutral position).

- Now to move in to cat pose.
- Exhale and draw your belly to your spine, rounding your back towards the ceiling. The pose should look like a cat stretching its back.
- Repeat for at least 5 breath cycles.

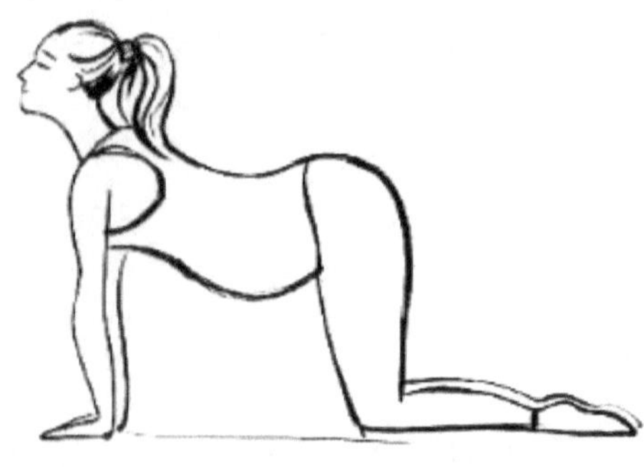

Cow Pose

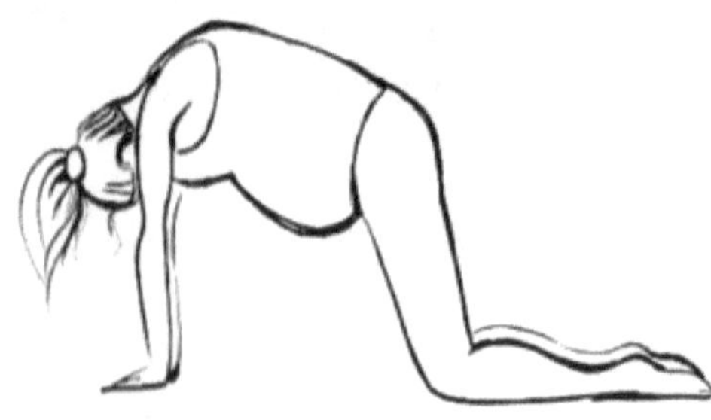

Cat Pose

This exercise helps to mobilise and strength the spine as well as the abdominal muscles.

Sleep

While some women may find that their sleep improves during the second trimester, others may experience mood swings, anxiety, or restless leg syndrome, all of which can affect sleep quality.

As your body changes to make space for your baby you may find it difficult to find a comfortable sleeping position, especially towards the end of the 2nd trimester. Sleeping on your side can cause tension in your hips so it is recommended to either use your duvet or a pregnancy pillow between your knees to keep your hips balanced and prevent lower back and pelvic discomfort.

Improving sleep during pregnancy is essential for the well-being of both you and your baby. Here are some tips to help you get better sleep:

- Stay Active: Engage in regular physical activity during the day, such as walking, swimming, or prenatal exercise classes, to help promote better sleep at night. Just be sure to avoid vigorous exercise close to bedtime, as it may energize you and make it harder to fall asleep.

- Watch Your Diet: Be mindful of what you eat and drink, especially in the hours leading up to bedtime. Avoid large meals, spicy foods, and caffeine, which can disrupt sleep. Instead, opt for light, soothing snacks and herbal teas.

- Stay Hydrated: Drink plenty of water throughout the day to stay hydrated, but try to limit your fluid intake in the evening to minimize nighttime bathroom trips.

- Establish a Bedtime Routine: Develop a relaxing bedtime routine to signal to your body that it's time to wind down. This could include activities like taking a warm bath, practicing gentle prenatal yoga, or reading a book. Maintain a consistent sleep schedule by going to bed and waking up at the same time each day, even on weekends. Avoid stimulating activities, such as watching TV or using electronic devices, close to bedtime, as the blue light can interfere with your ability to fall asleep.

- Create a Comfortable Sleep Environment: Make your bedroom conducive to sleep by keeping it cool, dark, and quiet. Invest in a comfortable mattress and pillows that support your growing body, and consider using blackout curtains or a white noise machine to block out any disturbances.

- Find a Comfortable Sleeping Position: Experiment with different sleeping positions to find one that is comfortable for you. Sleeping on your side with pillows supporting your abdomen and between your knees can help alleviate pressure on your back and hips. If you're experiencing discomfort while sleeping, such as back pain or heartburn, talk to your healthcare provider about strategies to manage these symptoms. They may recommend exercises, stretches, or over-the-counter remedies to help alleviate discomfort and improve sleep quality.

- Practice Relaxation Techniques: Incorporate relaxation techniques, such as deep breathing exercises, meditation, or progressive muscle relaxation, into your bedtime routine to help calm your mind and body before sleep.

- Seek Support: If you're struggling with sleep disturbances that persist despite trying these tips, don't hesitate to reach out to your healthcare provider for guidance and support. They can offer personalized recommendations and address any underlying issues that may be affecting your sleep.

Remember, prioritizing sleep during pregnancy is essential for your health and the health of your baby. By following these tips and making sleep a priority, you can improve your sleep quality and overall well-being during this special time.

Nutrition

Vitamin D

Nicknamed the "Sunshine Vitamin", Vitamin D is in fact a prohormone (substance which becomes a hormone). The body makes Vitamin D in a chemical reaction that occurs when sunlight hits the skin. This reaction produces cholecalciferol, and the liver converts it to calcidiol. The kidneys then convert the substance to calcitriol, which is the active form of the hormone in the body. Vitamin D helps regulate blood calcium concentration. Insufficient Vitamin D can impact immune system functions, increase the risk of cardiovascular disease, and mental illnesses.

Given the role of Vitamin D with calcium, too little during pregnancy can predispose the unborn child to rickets. Further to this recent research shows that taking large vitamin D during pregnancy can reduce the risk of complications, including gestational diabetes, preterm birth, infection, and might prevent pre-eclampsia.

According to WebMD:

Vitamin D supplementation is recommended during pregnancy and breast-feeding in daily amounts below 100mcg.

Vitamin D can help reduce the risk of complications, including gestational diabetes, preterm birth, and infection.

Foods containing high amounts of Vitamin D:

Portobello Mushrooms (exposed to UV or sunlight) - 13.1µg per 100g

Dehydrated Milk - 10.5µg per 100g

Dried eggs - 8.3µg per 100g

Chanterelle Mushrooms - 5.3µg per 100g

Morel Mushrooms - 5.1µg per 100g

Whole Milk 1.3µg per100g

Magnesium

Magnesium plays critical roles in immune, muscle, and nerve function. Deficiency during pregnancy may increase the risk of high blood pressure (hypertension) and premature labour.

Some studies suggest that supplementing with magnesium may reduce the risk of complications like chronic hypertension (pre-eclampsia), fetal growth restriction and preterm birth.

Magnesium can also be helpful with leg cramps as well as helping , a bath with two cups of Epsom salts (magnesium sulphate) can supplement your magnesium levels transdermally (absorbed through the skin) as well as the heat helping to relieve the muscles cramping.

According to WebMD:

Magnesium supplementation during pregnancy is recommended in daily amounts below 400mg.

Magnesium supplementation while breastfeeding is recommended in daily amounts below 360mg.

Magnesium can help reduce the risk of eclampsia and preterm birth.

Foods containing high amounts of magnesium:

Pumpkin seeds – 550mg per 100g

Almonds – 270mg per 100g

Dark chocolate – 228mg per 100g

Spinach – 87mg per 100g

Swiss chard – 86mg per 100g

Kale – 57mg per 100g

Protein

Proteins are found in every cell of the body. They provide structure to cells and help with their function as well as helping cells repair themselves. Protein is essential for the development of your baby's tissues and organs, making antibodies for their immune system and the transport of oxygen in the blood. It also necessary for both breast and uterine tissue growth for the mother.

According to WebMD:

The recommended daily intake of protein for pregnant and breast feeding women is 70mg.

Protein is essential for your baby's growth and can help reduce blood pressure complications.

Foods containing high amounts of protein:

Lean chicken breast – 32.1g per 100g

Non-fat mozzarella – 31.7g per 100g

Pumpkin seeds – 29.8g per 100g

Peanut butter – 24.1g per 100g

Almonds – 21.2g per 100g

Firm tofu – 17.3g per 100g

Part Three

The Third Trimester

The Third Trimester

"The moment a child is born,
the mother is also born."

\- Osho

Realising you are carrying a living being cannot be put in to words. For some it can be terrifying, for others its a realisation of how amazing the female body is. From around week 20 you will be able to feel the baby's movements, and by the start of the third trimester (week 29) the baby will start playing football with your bladder!

During this time you can feel tired as your body prioritises your baby's growth, however, it is still good to remain active where possible. Walking, pregnancy Pilates and yoga are three ways to exercise comfortably during the third trimester, but it is advised to consult your midwife if you have any current or previous pregnancy complications.

The third trimester is the preparation stage of pregnancy and while you are busy gathering the necessities for your new arrival it is also important to prepare yourself both mentally and physically.

If you haven't written your birth plan already, it is worth doing so now. This is talked about in the 2nd trimester, though there are various online resources available to help you begin. Further to this, your midwife should be well versed in birth plans so can also help!

Antenatal Activities

Tracking Movements

As your pregnancy progresses you will become more aware of your baby's movements. Keeping track of your baby's movements can help you notice any sudden increase, decrease or change in the way your baby moves.

Tommy's, the UK's largest pregnancy and baby loss charity, encourages movement tracking from week 16 onwards. Their campaign, Movement Matters, is backed by both the NHS and Kicks Count, and aims at educating families to prevent miscarriage and still birth.

According to Tommy's: women often hold back from reporting reduced movement for fear of 'wasting time' or 'being a nuisance'. Additionally it is common for women to wait for up to two days before reporting the changes to their midwife or doctor. This is primarily due to the lack of awareness on its importance.

Maternal intuition is now being studied in more depth. In a 2018 study, 84% of mothers who experienced a still birth had reported a "gut instinct" that something was wrong (Warland et al. 2017). Consequently, It is now being suggested that maternity care providers should be open to the possibility that maternal intuition begins in pregnancy, furthermore it may be unwise for them to discount the concerns of a pregnant mother about her unborn baby (Warland et al. 2017).

Bonding With Your Bump.

While preparing your home for your new arrival it is common to overlook your connection with the growing baby. It is beneficial for both parents and the baby to consider spending time bonding

with your bump!
Bonding with your bump can help form a healthier connection with your baby. This can also help prevent post-partum depression as well as relationship complications, as it allow both parents to form a connection in a positive affectionate manner.

Talking or Singing.

At 15 weeks your baby can hear sounds outside of the womb. By week 29, your babies can hear music and can recognise familiar voices. Regular vocal interaction with the bump will help the baby develop familiarity with your voices. Allocating regular quiet times to read stories, sing or even discuss general day to day plans with your bump allows both parents and baby to build a connection. Feeling your baby move and kick in response to your or your partner's voice can be very rewarding!

Massaging your Bump.

Another way to bond with your baby is through touch! Gentle stroking of your abdomen can create a gentle movement of your abdominal fluids, relaxing both yourself and the baby. This can be done by both parents too. Further in to the pregnancy you will be able to feel your .little one, as well as the occasional responsive kick or movement to your touch.
The use of oils or creams for stretch marks can be combined with your massage, keeping your skin moisturised and supple.

Pregnancy Massage.

Pregnancy massage is similar to normal massage but is adapted to maintain the well-being of the mother and her baby. Pregnancy massage, also known as prenatal massage, is a specialised form of massage therapy designed to support expectant mothers throughout all stages of pregnancy. It focuses on addressing the unique physical and emotional changes that occur during pregnancy, offering relief from discomfort such as lower back pain, swollen feet, and muscle tension. The massage techniques used are gentle and specifically tailored to accommodate the needs and safety considerations of pregnant women. Trained therapists understand the importance of positioning the mother-to-be comfortably and employing techniques that avoid pressure points that could potentially trigger contractions. Beyond the physical benefits, pregnancy massage provides a nurturing environment for relaxation, stress reduction, and emotional well-being, promoting a deeper connection between the mother and her growing baby. It can be a valuable part of prenatal care, offering you a moment of tranquility and rejuvenation during this transformative journey.

As with most antenatal treatments, pregnancy massage is considered safe after the first trimester, though it is worth consulting with your midwife or doctor beforehand, especially if you are experiencing complications or have a high risk of preterm labour.

Reported benefits of pregnancy massage are:

- Relief from pregnancy related muscle pains
- Reduced stress levels
- Improved energy
- Improved sleep

Obstetric Osteopathy

Osteopathy is an holistic manual therapy which uses various techniques to rebalance tensions throughout the body. Obstetric osteopathy is specialised to support the changes of pregnancy through releasing compressed joints while stabilising others, helping women maintain their mobility throughout their pregnancy. Obstetric osteopaths are able to examine and determine the causes of this, allowing them to formulate a gentle treatment to help relieve the pain and offer professional advice on how to maintain the effects of treatment and prevent recurrence. Obstetric osteopathy is a specialized branch of osteopathic medicine that focuses on the musculoskeletal health of pregnant women before, during, and after childbirth. Osteopathic practitioners who specialise in obstetrics aim to support women throughout the various stages of pregnancy, addressing musculoskeletal issues that may arise due to the physical changes and demands of pregnancy. These practitioners utilise a holistic approach, considering the interconnectedness of the body's systems and the impact that musculoskeletal imbalances can have on overall health and well-being during pregnancy. Techniques employed in obstetric osteopathy may include gentle manipulation, stretching, and soft tissue massage to alleviate discomfort, improve mobility, and promote optimal alignment of the pelvis and spine. By addressing musculoskeletal issues, obstetric osteopathy seeks to optimise the body's ability to adapt to the changes of pregnancy, potentially reducing the risk of complications during childbirth and enhancing overall maternal and fetal well-being. Additionally, obstetric osteopaths often provide guidance on posture, exercise, and self-care practices that can support women throughout their pregnancy journey. This approach aims to empower women with the tools and support they need to navigate the physical and emotional challenges of pregnancy and childbirth with greater ease and comfort.

Please consult your midwife or doctor if you are at risk of preterm labour, have a history or two or more miscarriages or are experiencing any complications.

Mental Health

As you approach the final hurdle of your journey it is common to experience unhelpful thoughts arising. Awareness of this change can help prevent the thoughts from becoming an ongoing issue. By now you will be starting to see your bump and this forces the realisation that you life is about to change. Considering how far you have come, in life and with your pregnancy juorney can help placate concerns but it is normal to feel apprehensive, especially if experiencing the negative stories from others as is an annoying 'side effect' of pregnancy.

Common antenatal concerns that Tommy's Pregnancy Hub notes:
- How will I cope with giving birth?
- Will my baby be OK?
- Will I be a good mother?
- Will this change my relationship with my partner?
- How will we manage for money?
- Can I go back to work or education afterwards?
- Will I still have a life of my own?
- Will a previous pregnancy problem happen again?
- Will something that I've done/eaten/drunk harm the baby?

Its understandable to worry about these things, especially if this is your first pregnancy, but it is advised to speak to your midwife, antenatal class or health advisor if these concerns affect your day to day mood and activities.

The UK now has a self referral system in place, though many aren't aware of this. It offers a few variations on therapy styles before an assessment is done. This service is faster than GP referral but is limited to 6 weeks at a time, with 6 month gaps between.

Relationship Changes

Other concerns can arise from a change a intimacy with your partner during pregnancy. As a result of powerful hormone changes, discomfort and other pregnancy related symptoms you may not wish to be as intimate as you have been previously. This is completely normal! Though it can in some cases it can be the polar opposite and this increased desire can also have an impact if your partner is not so willing.

Pregnancy is 9 months. It isn't forever. The changes will not stay this way, so try not to be too hard on yourself!

If your partner is being affected by pregnancy changes, it is worth reminding them that pregnancy isn't permanent.

Physical Changes

As the baby gains weight, your shape will change to accommodate this. Us women can be our own worst enemies and for many this change in shape can cause us to view ourselves negatively. As stated above, the change is not permanent and by taking care of yourself with mental health awareness, you can be realistic and appreciate the miraculous things your body is doing! In my personal experience, my figure became better after having my son. I felt more womanly and healthier as a result of this. While I know there are a fair few negative stories out there this doesn't mean they will be yours too! We naturally retain negative stories to protect ourselves, both a blessing and curse. However, the more you dwell on this the higher your cortisol levels will be. Cortisol affects are mentioned in the 2nd trimester.

Peer Support

Parents 1st UK are a charity that offers perinatal peer support for new families. Providing an invaluable contribution to healthier pregnancies and positive births. Many are reluctant to contact professionals to discuss difficulties so Parents 1st UK offers support from trained and supervised parents to help make it easier for new families to discuss their concerns without fear of judgement. The website to Parents 1st UK is included in the links section.

Post Partum Depression

As the saying goes: what goes up must come down, and this is the same with your physiology after labour.

For 9 months your body has worked flat out at 100%. Your body has peaked in immune function, nutritional absorption and tissue healing with the growth of your new arrival. At the end of this 9 months is labour and the start of a new learning curve with a small crying bundle of poop.

Your hormone levels will change significantly and while nursing so will your energy levels. Having a new baby on top of this can feel frustrating, especially while getting the little one in to a routine. There is no perfect way to parent, and all parents need to know this! Both you and the baby are learning together, so go easy on yourself and not expect miracles from yourself - no matter what you have been told by others. Further to this all children really are different! Your first may be hard work, it doesn't mean the rest will, and visa versa.

Every parenting journey is different and in some cases reading parenting books can help, but they can also make you see your journey negatively. There is no shame in asking for support or a little help from family and friends while you recover from labour and get yourself in the routine of parenting. There is no shame in asking for help when you are tired or worn out from sleepless nights. There is no shame in crying. Just know some days are harder than others and you are doing the best you can in the circumstances. We are often our own worst critic, but when we fell down learning to walk as a toddler, we got back up and carried on until we nailed it! Give yourself time to adapt and grow with your baby and you will have an easier time than if you put too much pressure on yourself!

Changes in the Third Trimester

Hormones

Oestrogen and progesterone both increase during the third trimester, peaking at around 32 weeks. Together they can help limit the release of stress hormones. Oestrogen is responsible for the synthesis of a water retention hormone and is thought to be involved in the increased swelling in hands and feet towards the end of the pregnancy. Progesterone can relax the cardiac sphincter of the stomach, increasing acid reflux significantly when paired with the increased pressure in the abdominal cavity.

Prolactin also increases in the 3rd trimester, by up to ten times the amount from the beginning of the pregnancy. This hormone stimulates the development of breast tissue preparing for lactation. You may begin to produce colostrum before labour and have the occasional leak from your nipples as a result.

Oxytocin is often considered the cuddle hormone but plays a vital role in female reproduction (Magon et al 2011). This hormone is believed to be increase significantly at the start of labour, along with a drop in progesterone. Oxytocin and oestrogen combine to release prostaglandins, which help soften the cervix in preparation for labour. Oxytocin also helps to eliminate the placenta post-labour by causing the required contractions. Doctors sometimes use a synthetic version called Pitocin to help induce labour.

Cavity Changes

During the third trimester the diaphragm is displaced upward, by up to 4cm from the neutral position. The rib cage widens and the sternum lifts forward in order to maintain lung capacity. Many mothers experience a severe shallowness of breath through this trimester (Lapinsky, 2016).

The intra-abdominal pressure increases as the uterus expands upwards. Towards the end of the pregnancy the uterus expands outwards, due to relaxation of the abdominal wall (Stone, 2007) and reduced fascial tensile strength. Pelvic organs are pushed further downwards.

Musculoskeletal Changes

The third trimester has the most rapid weight gain of the three trimesters, with the baby gaining up to 28g per day.

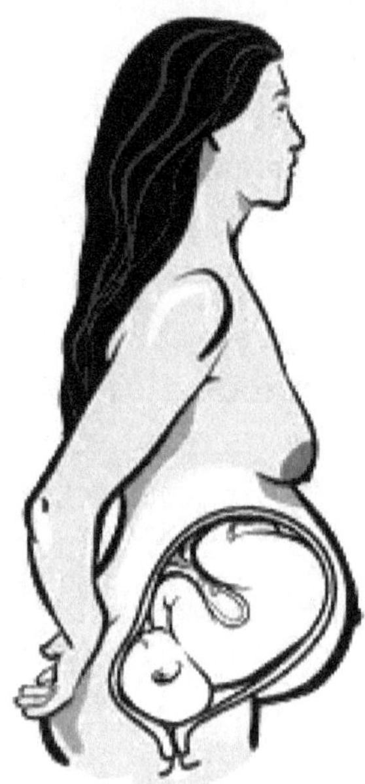

The overall spine can adapt in to either a lordotic or swayback posture.

The lordotic posture carries the majority of the uterus weight on the pubis (top of the anterior pelvis). This increases the pressure on the abdominal muscles, narrows the intervertebral spaces between the lumbar vertebrae and can result in strain at the lumbo-sacral junction of the spine (stone) and irritation on lumbar nerves, including the sciatic nerve. The anterior curve of the lumbar spine can increase up to 14.4 degrees from the neutral position (Kouhkan et al 2015).

The swayback posture carries the majority of the uterus weight on the pelvic floor, increasing tension in both the pelvic floor muscles and ligaments (Stone, 2007).

As the pregnancy progresses, your head angle can also change, as well as the position your head is carried. This anterior head carriage posture can result in hyperlordosis of the cervical spine and a strain on the cervico-dorsal junction (Stone, 2007), irritation of cervical nerves and tension headaches.

Carpal Tunnel Syndrome In Pregnancy

The carpal tunnel is narrow passageway surrounded by bones and ligaments on the palm side of your wrist. Carpal tunnel syndrome (CTS) is where the median nerve, which passes through the carpal tunnel is compressed or irritated, causing numbness and pain in the hands. The pain can occur in one or both hands and often begins at around week 30, where the most weight gain and fluid retention occurs (Christiano, 2018). There are variable factors which can increase the risk of developing CTS during pregnancy, these include:
  - Fluid retention
  - Hormone related joint swelling of the carpal bones
  - Gestational diabetes
  - Gestational hypertension (high blood pressure)

Stretching your wrists and the palms of your hands can help relieve the pressure in the carpal tunnel, helping prevent and reduce the symptoms of CTS.

Carpal Tunnel Wrist Stretches

Wrist Extension Stretch

Straighten your arm with your palm facing down without locking your elbow.

Bend your wrist upwards, palm facing out as if signalling someone to "stop".

Gently pull your hand towards you with the opposite hand until you feel a stretch in your wrist and forearm

Hold for 20 seconds.

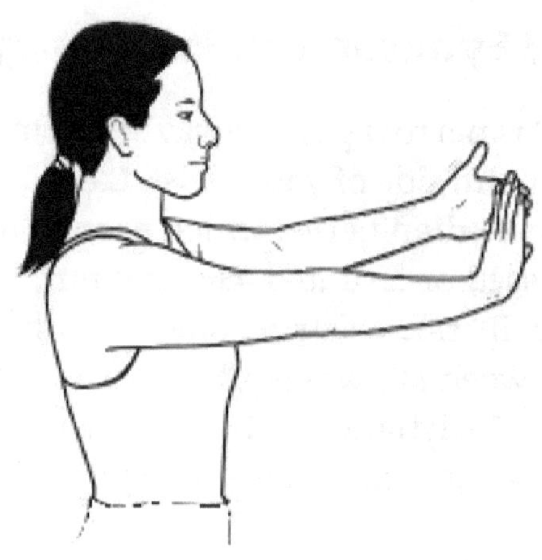

Wrist Flexion Stretch

Straighten your arm as above, remembering to not lock your elbow

Bend your wrist so that your fingers point downwards

Gently pull your hand towards you until you feel a stretch on the top of your forearm.

Hold for 20 seconds

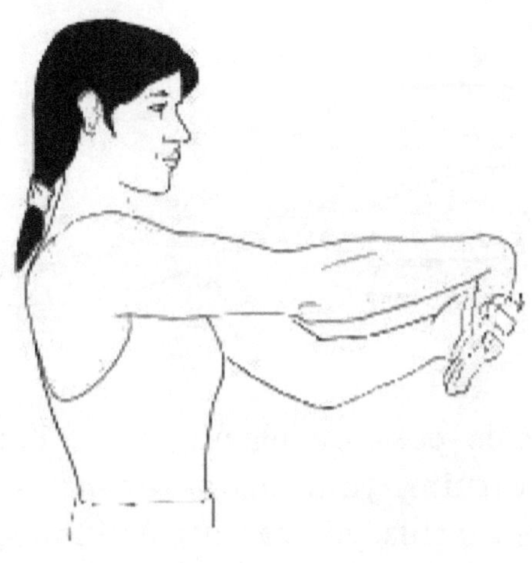

Back And Hip Pain Exercise

Child's Pose

Come on to your hands and knees.

Spread your knees as wide as your mat, keeping the tops of your feet on the floor with the big toes together.

Bring your bottom down toward your heels. Allowing your belly to rest between your thighs and rest your forehead on the floor or a yoga block.

Stretch your arms in front of your head, palms down, and allow your forearms to rest on the floor.

Hold for at least 20 seconds, but can be held for as long as you wish.

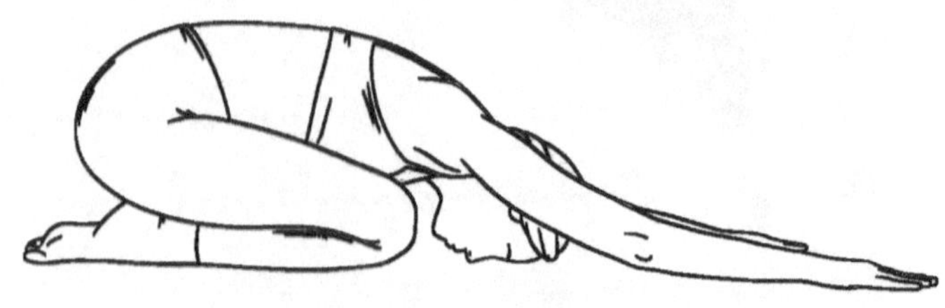

You can adapt this pose by placing your hands under your forehead or by turning your palms upwards to release your shoulders. Further to this, you can use a pillow under your chest and tummy to support your body and make this restful stretch more comfortable.

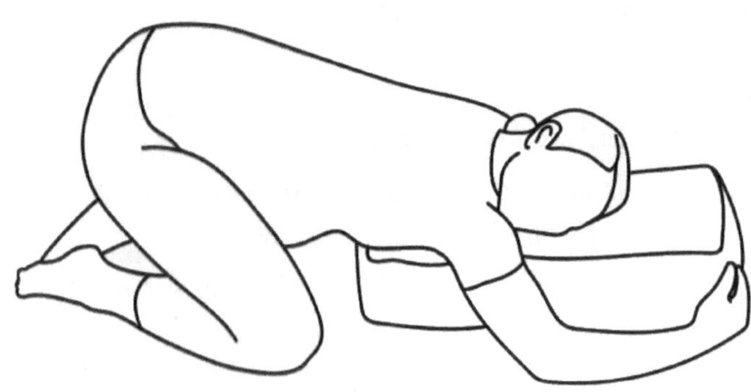

Hip Opening Exercise (32+ Weeks)

Deep Squat

NB: Please avoid this exercise if your baby is in a breech position or if you already are suffering with a prolapse as your pelvic floor muscles will be in a relaxed state doing this!

If unsure, you can use a chair to stabilise yourself as you lower yourself and a yoga block to support your pelvis. Only lower to a comfortable position. If you experience any pinching pains or discomfort please consult your midwife, GP or osteopath.

Stand with your feet shoulder width apart.

Have your feet turned outward slightly (find a position that is comfortable for your body).

Keep your chest up and lower your bottom to the floor.

Hold for 20 seconds.

Use your glutes (bottom muscles) to push yourself back up to standing.

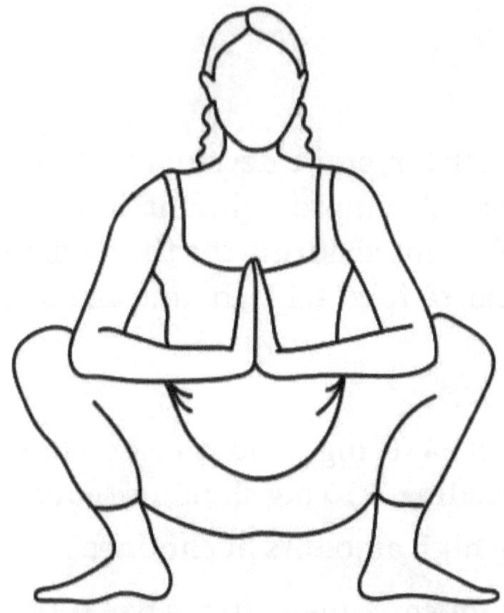

Nutrition

As with the previous two trimesters there are certain nutrients which can help support both yourself and the baby in the few weeks of pregnancy.

All of the nutritional data displayed here is taken from MyFoodData.com and is listed in order of highest amounts to lowest based on that shown on their database.

Choline

Choline is essential for brain development of the baby and is shown to significantly improve infant information processing speed when supplemented during the third trimester (Caudill, M., et al 2018). Similar to folic acid, choline can also prevent neural tube defects.

According to WebMD:

When pregnant, 450 mg should be consumed daily, and when breast-feeding, 550 mg should be consumed daily.

Foods containing high amounts of choline:

Dried shiitake mushrooms – 201mg per 100g

Lean chicken breast – 117mg per 100g

Salmon (wild caught) – 112.6mg per 100g

Sun dried tomatoes – 84.3mg per 100g

Oyster mushrooms – 48.7 per 100g

Broccoli – 40.1mg per 100g

Vitamin K2

Vitamin K2 (Menaquinone) has only recently emerged on research scene, previously considered to be a variant of K1 which is essential for blood clotting. Vitamin K2 is responsible for activation of osteocalcin, which directs calcium from the bloodstream to bones and teeth, keeping them strong and healthy. In pregnancy this can help prevent pregnancy related osteoporosis promote cardiovascular health (prevention of vascular calcification), and improves bone formation and mineralisation for both mother and baby.

According to FutureYou Cambridge:

Adults should ensure they are getting between 100 and 300 micrograms of vitamin K2 per day

There are no known serious side effects from taking too much vitamin K2. However, it is sensible to stick to the recommended intake.

Foods containing high amounts of Vitamin K2:

Natto (Fermented soybeans) – 1000μg per 100g

Jarlsberg – 73μg per 100g

Gouda – 73μg per 100g

Pepperoni – 41.7μg per 100g

Chicken Drumsticks – 35.7μg per 100g

Salami – 28μg per 100g

Omega-3

Omega-3s are essential fatty acids with anti-inflammatory properties which are associated with reducing the risk of preterm birth and pre-eclampsia in pregnancy (Middleton et al 2018). Essential fatty acids are lipids that cannot be synthesized within the body and must be ingested through the diet or from supplements (Colleta et al 2010). The richest sources of these omega-3 fatty acids are marine sources, such as seafood and fish oil supplements, however certain species of fish contain higher levels of mercury and pregnant women are advised to avoid consumption of these fish (Colleta et al 2010). Docosahexaenoic Acid (DHA) is a biologically active omega-3 fatty acid found in fish and seafood. DHA is has a key role eye and nerve development as well as reducing inflammation. DHA can be converted from Alpha Linolenic Acids (ALA) in the body. The rate of ALA to DHA conversion is poor in humans and can result in excess unconverted ALA being stored for energy with other fats. ALA is commonly found in plant based foods.

According to Healthline:

200 mg of DHA is recommended during pregnancy and breastfeeding

Omega-3 fatty acids, especially DHA, are vital before, during, and after pregnancy

Foods containing high amounts of Omega-3:

Walnuts – 9080mg per 100g

Salmon – 2501mg per 100g

Anchovies – 1303mg per 100g

Firm Tofu – 582mg per 100g

Brussels sprouts – 173mg per 100g

Avocado – 111mg per 100g

Labour

By now you may have looked in to your antenatal classes and had one or more scans of your baby. Your health advisor or midwife will have, at the very least, given you an outline of the labour process; braxton hicks, contractions, dilation and pushing, but very little detail about what actually happens at each of these stages, what to expect and what to do. More often than not the information you are given can make you feel anxious, even more so as the due date approaches and you feel unprepared for labour. This chapter discusses what your body is doing at each stage of labour as well as afterward and the various ways that you may experience these stages.

There are numerous tips to help prepare you but this will vary from one health professional to the next. Raspberry leaf tea from 32 weeks onwards is said to help reduce complications in labour by toning the muscles in the uterus. Chilli sauce (serious spicy chilli, not sweet chilli) helped my son arrive a day early (6 hours after consumption) and helped a tutor's overdue wife. That being said it might not work for everyone else. These are just two things I do recommend, however it is worth discussing with your health professional or midwife before you try them yourself.

Stages Of Labour

Hopefully by this point you have attended antenatal classes at the very least and have an idea of how you wish to proceed. Regardless of this it's still worth outlining each stage so you have a better idea of what to expect. There are various pain relief options available depending on your circumstances. Please remember this is your labour so the choices are yours, if you wish to be up and active then do so!

Braxton Hicks

Braxton-Hicks (BH) contractions are contractions of the uterus that can be felt as early as in the second trimester and are often referred to as false labour pains. The main difference in BH contractions and labour contractions is the level of discomfort as well as frequency of the pains, BH being considerably less in both. These contractions are the body's way of preparing for labour though not all experience them. The discomfort can present as a stomach cramp, similar to trapped wind, or lower back ache. Placing a hot water bottle on the affected area can help reduce the discomfort.

Stage 1 of Labour: Dilation
This is often the longest of the four stages of labour and is divided in to 3 phases: the early phase, the active phase and the transitional phase.

The early phase begins with contractions occurring from 20 minutes to as little as 5 minutes apart and lasting 30 to 60 seconds each. The contractions can begin feeling like BH but intensify as they become more frequent. As with BH, heat can help control the discomfort so women are often advised to have a bath while waiting for the contractions to become more frequent. These contractions are your cervix dilating, in preparation for the baby to pass through.

You may see a pink jelly discharge, called show, which is the mucus plug that blocks the cervical opening during pregnancy. The show is a strong indicator or labour, as is the rupture of the foetal membranes, commonly known as water breaking. If there is vaginal bleeding or you feel unsure about anything please call your doctor or maternity department so they can advise you, it is their job after all!

When your cervix has dilated to around 3cm the active phase begins. During this phase the contractions become stronger and more frequent, occurring every 2 - 3 minutes. Your cervix is dilating faster and you will have less rest time between. Your cervix will continue to open until around 8cm. This size allows the baby's head to begin descending further in to the pelvis. If it hasn't already, your water may break at this stage. Further to this, you may feel lower back pressure on top of the increasing contractions.

Around this time you may feel the urge to sit on the toilet or squat, this is quite common! If you have a large gym ball, feel free to sit on this if it helps or try various positions that make you feel as comfortable as possible during the contractions.

The transitional phase is the final phase for cervical dilation, where it will expand up to 10cm, which is ideal for the baby to pass through. At this stage the contractions will occur every 2 - 3 minutes, lasting up to 60 seconds. You may feel unsteady and nauseous at this point as the baby descends further in to the pelvis. By the end of this phase a birth canal will have formed. This is a passage from the womb, through the cervix to the vagina allowing the baby to pass through.

Stage 2 of Labour: Delivery

This stage begins once the cervix is fully dilated to 10cm. The contractions occur every 1 to 3 minutes and last up to 75 seconds. As each contraction increases you may feel the urge to bear down and push.

Your midwife or doctor may ask you to push, helping the baby through the birth canal.

Pushing or bearing down is best described as an action similar to passing a stool when constipated. Breathing techniques, such as Lamaze, can help during this stage.

Crowning is where he baby's head emerges at the opening of the vagina, working to stretch out the vagina. Once the baby's head has been delivered, the shoulders and body will follow.

Stage 3 of Labour: Afterbirth

After the baby is born the third stage of labour begins and ends with pushing out the placenta. This can occur between 5 to 30 minutes after childbirth and in many cases is induced by your doctor.

Contractions help the placenta separate from the uterus wall. You may be asked to push again by your doctor or midwife as they use the umbilical cord to encourage the placenta out.

Stage 4 of Labour: Recovery
This begins during the first 2 to 3 hours after delivery with the uterus contracting to push out anything remaining inside and regain muscle tone.

You may feel discomfort from the labour as well as tremors or chills at this stage but it varies as many women can feel quite energetic after labour as a result of endorphins. Only do what you feel comfortable doing during this time, your partner can assist with skin to skin contact if you do not feel up to it.

As with pregnancy, every labour is different. The more you are prepared with antenatal activities the less stressful this stage will be. Your body is more amazing than you know and from personal experience I am certain that you will begin to see this once you have had your baby.

Part Four

The Fourth Trimester

The Fourth Trimester

"Postpartum is a quest back to yourself. Alone in your body again. You will never be the same, you are stronger than you were."

\- Amethyst Joy

The fourth trimester is the 12 weeks following the birth of your baby. Not everyone has heard of it, but every parent and their newborn baby will experience it. It is a time of great physical and emotional change as your baby adjusts to being outside the womb, and you adjust to your new life as a parent.

Planning your fourth trimester can be just as beneficial as planning the birth if not more so, as this can help reduce the risk of post-partum depression (PPD).

Planning for the fourth trimester, often referred to as the postpartum period, is a crucial aspect of pregnancy that is sometimes overshadowed by the focus on childbirth itself. This transitional phase, lasting roughly three months after giving birth, is a time of immense change and adjustment for both mother and baby. Central to this planning process is prioritizing maternal well-being, both physically and emotionally. Establishing a care plan that includes ample rest, proper nutrition, and support from healthcare professionals and loved ones is essential for promoting optimal recovery and preventing complications. Moreover, anticipating and preparing for the challenges of breastfeeding, if chosen, or alternative feeding methods, can help ease the transition into motherhood. Creating a nurturing environment at home, conducive to bonding and relaxation, is also crucial during this period. This may involve arranging for practical support with household chores and childcare duties, allowing the new mother to focus on her own recovery and adjusting to her new role. Additionally, planning for postpartum mental health support is vital, as many women experience a range of emotions during this time, including the "baby blues" or more serious conditions like postpartum depression. Having access to resources such as support groups, therapy, or counseling can provide essential emotional support and guidance during this period of adjustment. Lastly, involving partners and family members in the planning process fosters a sense of teamwork and shared responsibility, strengthening familial bonds and ensuring a smoother transition into parenthood. In essence, planning for the fourth trimester encompasses a holistic approach that addresses physical, emotional, and practical aspects, laying the groundwork for a positive experience for both mother and baby.

Breast, Bottle or Both?

Whether this is your first pregnancy or third, it is your choice to breastfeed, use bottles or both when feeding your baby. All options come with their own set of benefits. Breastfeeding offers numerous advantages, including providing optimal nutrition tailored to your baby's needs, as breast milk contains essential nutrients, antibodies, and enzymes that support your baby's growth and development. Breastfeeding also promotes bonding between you and your baby through skin-to-skin contact and helps establish a strong emotional connection. Additionally, breastfeeding has been associated with a lower risk of certain health conditions for both mother and baby, such as reduced risk of infections for the baby and decreased risk of breast and ovarian cancer for the mother. On the other hand, using bottles allows for greater flexibility and convenience, as it allows other caregivers to feed the baby and provides the option of using formula if breastfeeding is not possible or preferred. Bottle-feeding can also help ensure that the baby receives adequate nutrition and allows for precise measurement of intake. Ultimately, this decision depends on your individual circumstances and preferences but never feel pressured in to doing anything that doesn't work for you and your baby!

Feeding Positions

Cradle Hold

The cradle hold breastfeeding position is one of the most common and widely practiced techniques among nursing mothers. In this position, the baby lies horizontally across the mother's body, with their head resting in the crook of her arm, while their body is supported by her forearm and hand. The mother can use her free hand to support her breast and guide the baby's mouth to latch onto the 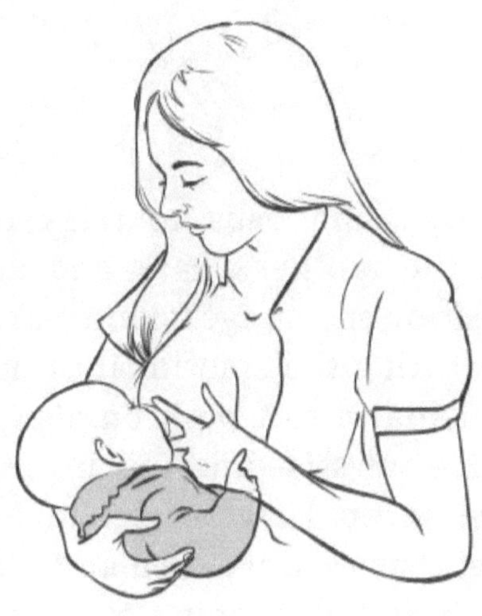 nipple. The cradle hold allows for close eye contact between mother and baby, promoting bonding and facilitating communication during feeding sessions. Additionally, this position can be comfortable for many mothers, as it allows them to sit upright or recline slightly while breastfeeding. However, it's important for mothers to ensure proper positioning and latch to prevent nipple pain or discomfort. Overall, the cradle hold breastfeeding position offers a combination of comfort, intimacy, and convenience for both mother and baby during feeding sessions.

Side Lying

The side lying breastfeeding position offers a comfortable and convenient option for nursing mothers, especially during

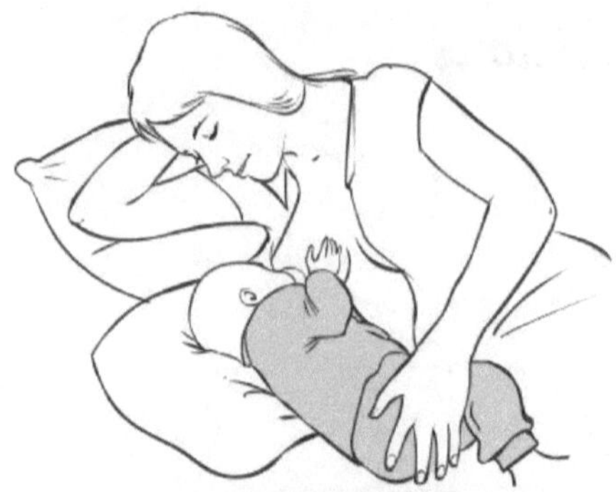

nighttime feedings or moments when they need to rest. In this position, the mother lies on her side, with her baby positioned facing her chest. The baby can latch onto the breast while lying on their side, with their body aligned parallel to the mother's. This position allows both mother and baby to relax fully, as there is minimal strain on the mother's back and arms. Additionally, the side lying position encourages skin-to-skin contact, promoting bonding and nurturing the emotional connection between mother and baby. Nursing in this position also allows mothers to easily doze off while breastfeeding, making nighttime feedings less disruptive to their sleep. However, it's important for mothers to ensure that their baby's airway remains clear and that they maintain proper latch and positioning to prevent any discomfort or issues with breastfeeding. Overall, the side lying breastfeeding position offers a comfortable and intimate way for mothers to nourish their babies while also promoting rest and relaxation for both.

Laid Back

The laid-back breastfeeding position, also known as biological nurturing hold, offers a relaxed approach to breastfeeding. In this position, the mother reclines comfortably while her baby is placed tummy-down on her chest. This positioning allows gravity to assist the baby in latching onto the breast, often without much assistance from the mother. The laid-back position encourages babies to use their innate reflexes to seek out the breast, promoting a deep latch and effective milk transfer. Moreover, the relaxed posture of the mother encourages skin-to-skin contact and facilitates bonding between mother and baby. This position is particularly beneficial for newborns and infants with difficulties latching or for mothers recovering from childbirth, as it minimizes strain on the mother's body and allows for comfortable and stress-free breastfeeding sessions. Overall, the laid-back breastfeeding position provides a natural and nurturing approach to breastfeeding that supports both the physical and emotional needs of mother and baby alike.

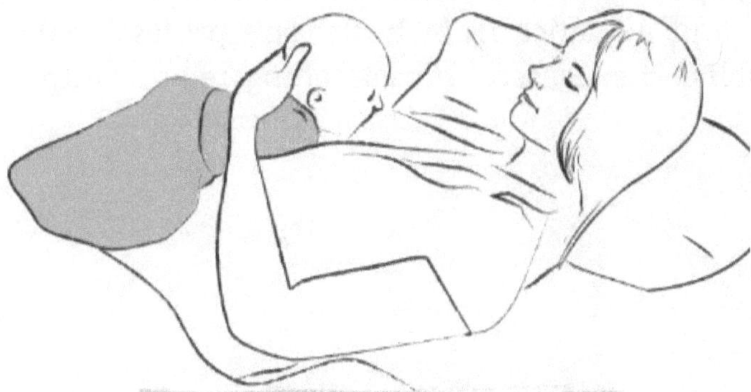

You will find there are positions that work better for you than others, and some better depending on the cirsumstances. The side lying position is great for the first feed of the day and allows you to relax in bed while your baby feeds!

There are more positions and variations of the positions I have included but these three are a great start for you to have a go at.

Latching

Latching refers to the way a baby attaches to the mother's breast to nurse effectively. A proper latch ensures that the baby is able to extract milk efficiently while preventing nipple pain or damage for the mother. A good latch involves the baby taking a large mouthful of breast tissue, with the nipple and much of the areola (the darker area around the nipple) in their mouth. This ensures that the baby is able to compress the milk ducts and stimulate milk flow effectively. Achieving a good latch requires proper positioning of both mother and baby, with the baby's mouth wide open and lips flanged outward, creating a seal around the breast. Additionally, it's important for the baby to have a deep latch, meaning their tongue is positioned below the nipple and areola, allowing them to draw milk from the breast efficiently. A proper latch not only facilitates effective milk transfer but also reduces the risk of nipple soreness and encourages the release of oxytocin, promoting bonding between mother and baby. Latching is a skill that may take time and practice to master, but with patience, support, and guidance from healthcare professionals, mothers can establish a successful breastfeeding relationship with their babies.

Changes during the Fourth Trimester

During the fourth trimester, the first three months after childbirth, the body undergoes several physical changes as it adjusts to postnatal recovery and the demands of caring for a newborn. Some of the main physical changes during this period include:

- Uterine Involution: After childbirth, the uterus undergoes a process called involution, where it gradually returns to its pre-pregnancy size and shape. This process involves the shedding of excess uterine tissue and the contraction of uterine muscles, which helps to control bleeding and promote healing. This can take up to six weeks to complete and you may experience cramps (called afterpains) during uterine involution.

- Vaginal Bleeding (Lochia): In the days and weeks following childbirth, you may experience vaginal bleeding known as lochia. Lochia consists of blood, mucus, and uterine tissue and is a normal part of the postnatal recovery process. The flow of lochia gradually decreases over time and may transition from bright red to pink or brownish in colour.

- Perineal Healing: If you had a vaginal delivery or episiotomy, your perineum (the area between the vagina and anus) may be swollen, bruised, or sore after childbirth. Perineal healing occurs as the tissues repair themselves, and discomfort typically improves with time.

- Breast Changes: The breasts undergo significant changes during the fourth trimester as they prepare for breastfeeding. Initially, breasts may become engorged, swollen, and tender as milk production begins. Over time, engorgement typically resolves as breastfeeding establishes a regular milk supply. Women may also experience changes in breast size, shape, and sensitivity as hormonal fluctuations occur.

- Abdominal Changes: The abdomen undergoes gradual changes during the fourth trimester as it returns to its pre-pregnancy state. Women may experience abdominal cramping or discomfort as the uterus contracts (see uterine involution). Abdominal muscles may also feel weak or stretched, particularly if they separated during pregnancy (diastasis recti). Engaging in gentle abdominal exercises and wearing supportive clothing may help promote abdominal muscle recovery.

- Hormonal Fluctuations: Hormonal fluctuations continue to occur during the fourth trimester as the body adjusts to the changes associated with childbirth and lactation. These hormonal changes can affect mood, energy levels, and physical symptoms such as hot flashes or night sweats.

  NB: the significant drop in pregnancy hormones has been linked to PPD symptoms, so being aware of this change and understanding that a low mood is likely caused by our incredibly powerful endocrines can make a big difference in your recovery process.

- Sleep: Caring for a newborn often leads to disrupted sleep patterns during the fourth trimester. Sleep deprivation, coupled with adjusting to a new routine, can result in fatigue which may impact overall well-being.

Overall, the fourth trimester is a period of significant physical adjustment as the body transitions from pregnancy to postnatal recovery. While some physical changes are temporary and resolve with time, others may require medical attention or support from healthcare providers to promote healing and well-being.

Preparing for postnatal recovery is essential for ensuring a smooth transition after childbirth. Here are some tips to help you prepare:

Support

Arranging support from your partner, family members, or friends for the first few weeks after childbirth is essential prior to giving birth.

Having someone to help with household chores, meal preparation, and caring for the baby can give you the rest and recuperation you need.

Postnatal support, encompassing both practical assistance and emotional encouragement, plays a vital role in the well-being of new mothers and their babies. By providing help with daily tasks such as cooking, cleaning, and caring for the newborn, postnatal support allows mothers to focus on their own recovery while nurturing their babies. Additionally, emotional support from partners, family members, or friends can ease the transition into motherhood, offering reassurance, companionship, and a listening ear during this transformative period. Benefits of postnatal support include faster physical recovery, reduced risk of PPD, enhanced bonding with the baby, and encouragement of self-care practices. Ultimately, by fostering a nurturing environment and alleviating the burdens of new parenthood, postnatal support empowers mothers to thrive as they embark on their journey of motherhood.

Planning for postnatal support is crucial for several reasons:

- Physical Recovery: Childbirth is physically demanding, and the postnatal period is a time when your body needs rest and care to heal. Having support means you can delegate tasks like cooking, cleaning, and running errands, allowing you to focus on recuperating.

- Emotional Well-being: The postnatal period can be emotionally challenging due to hormonal changes, sleep deprivation, and adjusting to the demands of caring for a newborn. Having emotional support from partners, family members, or friends can provide comfort, reassurance, and someone to talk to during this transition.

- Bonding with Baby: Postnatal support can also help facilitate bonding with your newborn. When you have assistance with tasks like diaper changes, feeding, and soothing, you can devote more time and energy to connecting with your baby and enjoying those early moments together.

- Breastfeeding Support: If you choose to breastfeed, having support from lactation consultants, experienced mothers, or healthcare providers can be invaluable. They can offer guidance, tips, and troubleshooting advice to help you establish and maintain successful breastfeeding.

- Promotes Recovery: Adequate support during the postnatal period can contribute to a smoother and faster recovery overall. By reducing stress, ensuring proper nutrition, and promoting rest, support can help prevent complications and promote healing.

- Reduces Risk of Post-partum Depression: Having a strong support system in place can reduce the risk of post-partum depression and anxiety. Knowing that you have people you can rely on for practical help and emotional support can provide a buffer against feelings of isolation and overwhelm.

- Encourages Self-Care: When you have support, you're more likely to prioritize self-care, which is essential for your physical and mental well-being. Taking time for yourself to rest, shower, or engage in activities you enjoy can help prevent burnout and support your overall recovery.

Planning for support is essential for ensuring that you have the resources and assistance you need to navigate the challenges of the post-partum period, promote healing, and adjust to life with a new baby. Hormonal changes after childbirth can trigger a range of emotions some harder to manage than others. Stay connected with loved ones, and don't hesitate to seek professional help if you're struggling emotionally.

NB: It's okay to accept help from others, whether it's with household chores, childcare, or emotional support. Trying to do everything yourself can lead to burnout and delay the recovery process.

Nutrition

Nutrition during the fourth trimester is just as important as the previous three trimesters. This period is marked by significant physical and emotional changes as you recover from childbirth, adjust to breastfeeding (if chosen to do so), and navigate the demands of caring for a newborn. Proper nutrition during this time is essential for supporting your postnatal recovery, replenishing nutrient stores depleted during pregnancy and childbirth, and promoting overall health and well-being. Nutrient-rich foods provide the energy and nutrients needed for tissue repair, wound healing, and the production of breast milk should you choose to breast feed. Additionally, adequate nutrition supports maternal mental health by providing nutrients that support brain function and mood regulation, helping to alleviate symptoms of postnatal mood disorders such as anxiety and depression. Proper nutrition also supports hormonal balance, which continues to fluctuate during the postnatal period as your body adjusts to the cessation of pregnancy hormones and the initiation of lactation.

As I have covered a vast amount of nutrition in the previous parts I will give an overview for your recovery nutrition, please feel free to go back to allocate food that work better for you from each of these food groups!

Here are some foods that are beneficial for postnatal recovery:

- Lean Protein: Foods like lean meats, poultry, fish, eggs, tofu, and legumes are rich in protein, which is essential for repairing tissues and supporting muscle recovery after childbirth.

- Fruits and Vegetables: Colourful fruits and vegetables provide vitamins, minerals, antioxidants, and fibre that support overall health and help replenish nutrients lost during childbirth. Aim for a variety of fruits and vegetables to ensure you're getting a wide range of nutrients.

- Whole Grains: Whole grains like oats, quinoa, brown rice, and whole wheat provide complex carbohydrates, fibre, and essential nutrients such as iron and B vitamins. These nutrients help replenish energy stores and support healthy digestion.

- Healthy Fats: Incorporate sources of healthy fats, such as avocados, nuts, seeds, and fatty fish like salmon, into your diet. Healthy fats are important for hormone production, brain function, and overall cellular health.

- Dairy or Calcium-Rich Foods: Calcium is important for bone health, especially during the postnatal period when your body may be recovering from pregnancy and childbirth. Include dairy products like milk, yogurt, and cheese, as well as calcium-fortified plant-based alternatives, in your diet.

- Iron-Rich Foods: Iron is crucial for replenishing iron stores depleted during pregnancy and childbirth, as well as supporting energy levels and preventing anaemia. Include iron-rich foods such as lean meats, poultry, fish, fortified cereals, legumes, and dark leafy greens.

- Hydrating Foods: Staying hydrated is important for postnatal recovery and breastfeeding. Incorporate hydrating foods like water-rich fruits and vegetables (e.g., watermelon, cucumber, oranges) into your diet, along with plenty of fluids like water, herbal teas, and broths.

- Foods Rich in Omega-3 Fatty Acids: Omega-3 fatty acids, found in fatty fish, flaxseeds, chia seeds, and walnuts, have anti-inflammatory properties and support brain health. Including these foods in your diet may help reduce inflammation and support mood during the postnatal period.

- Herbs and Spices: Some herbs and spices, such

as ginger and turmeric, have anti-inflammatory properties and may help reduce postnatal discomfort and inflammation. Certain herbal supplements like fenugreek can help with breast milk production as well as recovery. It is worth discussing these with a registered herbalist and your midwife to find what is best for you.

Eating a balanced diet that includes a variety of nutrient-dense foods will not only support your postnatal recovery but can also provide nutritional benefits for your baby. Be sure to consult with your healthcare provider or a registered dietitian for personalized nutrition advice based on your individual needs and any specific dietary considerations.

Gentle Exercise

While it's important to rest, gentle exercise can help improve circulation, boost energy levels, and promote faster healing.

I cannot do diret recommendations on this section as you will need to have exercises ailored to your needs and circumstances, but the diaphragm breathing (in part one) and pelvic tilts (in part two are commonly used to assist in the healing process.

Starting with light activities like walking and gradually adding post natal specific exercises such as postnatal yoga allows you increase intensity as you feel ready. Strengthening your pelvic floor muscles can help prevent urinary incontinence and improve overall pelvic health. Ask your healthcare provider about recommended exercises, such as Kegels to assist you with this.

Afterword

Congratulations! You've reached the conclusion of this self-help guide on navigating the beautiful journey of pregnancy. As you reflect on the insights gained throughout this book, remember that the essence of pregnancy lies in your personal preferences! Throughout these pages, we've delved into various aspects of pregnancy, and things you can add to make the journey more enjoyable. I hope this book has helped you learn to embrace the changes and challenges that come with each trimester, finding strength and resilience within yourself while doing so.

But this journey isn't just about the destination; it's about the experiences, the growth, and the connections forged along the way. As you prepare to embark on the adventure of parenthood, remember to cherish every moment, from feeling the flutter of your baby's first kicks to marveling at the miracle of birth.

As you navigate the ups and downs of pregnancy, remember to prioritize self-care and nurture your well-being, both physically and emotionally. Surround yourself with a supportive network of loved ones, healthcare professionals, and fellow mothers who can offer guidance, encouragement, and understanding.

Above all, trust in yourself and your body's innate wisdom to carry you through this incredible journey. You are stronger, more capable, and more resilient than you realize. Embrace the changes, celebrate the milestones, and savour the moments of joy and anticipation that pregnancy brings.

As you turn the final page of this book, know that you are embarking on one of the most transformative and rewarding experiences of your life. Embrace the journey, trust in yourself, and cherish the miracle of new life growing within you. You've got this, mama!

References

Bermas, B., Lockwood, C. and Eckler, K. (2017). Musculoskeletal changes and pain duringpregnancy and postpartum. [online] Uptodate.com. Available at:<https://www.uptodate.com/contents/musculoskeletal-changes-and-pain-during-pregnancy-and-postpartum/> [Accessed 29 March 2021].

Betz D, Fane K. Human Chorionic Gonadotropin. [Updated 2023 Aug 14]. In: StatPearls [Internet]. Treasure Island (FL): StatPearls Publishing; 2023 Jan-. Available from: https://www.ncbi.nlm.nih.gov/books/NBK532950/

Caudill, M., Strupp, B., Muscalu, L., Nevins, J., & Canfield, R. (2018). Maternal choline supplementation during the third trimester of pregnancy improves infant information processing speed: a randomized, double-blind, controlled feeding study. The FASEB Journal, 32(4), 2172-2180. https://doi.org/10.1096/fj.201700692rr

Coletta, J. M., Bell, S. J., & Roman, A. S. (2010). Omega-3 Fatty acids and pregnancy. Reviews in obstetrics & gynecology, 3(4), 163–171.

Conder, R., Zamani, R. and Akrami, M., 2019. The Biomechanics of Pregnancy: A Systematic Review. Journal of Functional Morphology and Kinesiology, 4(4), p.72.

Dennis, C., Falah-Hassani, K. and Shiri, R., 2017. Prevalence of antenatal and postnatal anxiety: Systematic review and meta-analysis. *British Journal of Psychiatry*, 210(5), pp.315-323.

Greenberg JA, Bell SJ, Guan Y, Yu YH. Folic Acid supplementation and pregnancy: more than just neural tube defect prevention. *Reviews in Obstetric Gynecololgy* 2011 Summer;4(2):52-9. PMID:

22102928; PMCID: PMC3218540.

Heazell, A., Warland, J., Stacey, T., Coomarasamy, C., Budd, J., Mitchell, E., & O'Brien, L. (2017). Stillbirth is associated with perceived alterations in fetal activity – findings from an international case control study. *BMC Pregnancy And Childbirth*, 17(1). https://doi.org/10.1186/s12884-017-1555-6

Hinkle, S., Mumford, S., Grantz, K., Silver, R., Mitchell, E., Sjaarda, L., Radin, R., Perkins, N., Galai, N. and Schisterman, E., 2016. Association of Nausea and Vomiting During Pregnancy With Pregnancy Loss. *JAMA Internal Medicine*, 176(11), p.1621.

Kouhkan, S., Rahimi, A., Ghasemi, M., Naimi, S. and Baghban, A., 2015. Postural Changes during First Pregnancy. *British Journal of Medicine and Medical Research*, 7(9), pp.744-753.

Lapinsky, S. (2016). Pregnancy. *Thoracic Key*. Retrieved 4 December 2021, from https://thoracickey.com/pregnancy/.

Law R, Maltepe C, Bozzo P, Einarson A. (2010). Treatment of heartburn and acid reflux associated with nausea and vomiting during pregnancy. *Canadian Family Physician*. 2010 Feb;56(2):143-4. PMID: 20154244; PMCID: PMC2821234.

Lu, H., Zheng, C., Zhong, Y., Cheng, L. and Zhou, Y., 2021. Effectiveness of Acupuncture in the Treatment of Hyperemesis Gravidarum: A Systematic Review and Meta-Analysis. *Evidence-Based Complementary and Alternative Medicine*, 2021, pp.1-14.

Masson GM, Anthony F, Chau E. Serum chorionic gonadotropin (hCG), schwangerschafts protein 1 (SP1), progesterone, and oestradiol levels in patients with nausea and vomiting in early pregnancy. *British Journal of Obstetric Gynaecology* 1985;92:211–215.

Magon, N., & Kalra, S. (2011). The orgasmic history of oxytocin: Love, lust, and labor. *Indian Journal Of Endocrinology And Metabolism*, 15(7), 156. https://doi.org/10.4103/2230-8210.84851

Mei, Q., Gu, Y. and Fernandez, J. (2018). Alterations of Pregnant Gait during Pregnancy and Post-Partum. *Scientific Reports*, 8(1).

Middleton, P., Gomersall, J., Gould, J., Shepherd, E., Olsen, S., & Makrides, M. (2018). Omega-3 fatty acid addition during pregnancy. *Cochrane Database Of Systematic Reviews, 2018*(11). https://doi.org/10.1002/14651858.cd003402.pub3

Mittal, R. (1998). How can the sphincteric action of the diaphragm in humans be described?-What is the relationship between contraction at the esophagogastric junction and increase inintra-abdominal pressure?. [online] Oeso.org. Available at:<http://www.oeso.org/OESO/books/Vol_5_Eso_Junction/Articles/art004.html>[Accessed29 March 2021].

Novakovic, A., 2017. Morning sickness: Treatments, prevention, and when it starts. [online]Medicalnewstoday.com. Available at:<https://www.medicalnewstoday.com/articles/179633>[Accessed 29 March 2021].

Schlessinger, D., Anoruo, M. and Schlessinger, J. (2021). Biochemistry, Melanin. [online] Ncbi.nlm.nih.gov. Available at: <https://www.ncbi.nlm.nih.gov/books/NBK459156/> [Accessed 19 August 2021].

Stone, C. (2007). Visceral and obstetric osteopathy. Edinburgh: Churchill Livingston/Elsevier.

Vazquez J. C. (2015). Heartburn in pregnancy. *BMJ clinical evidence*, 2015, 1411.

www.ingramcontent.com/pod-product-compliance
Lightning Source LLC
Chambersburg PA
CBHW031312250726
48656CB00005B/1754